Note of Devotion

To,

Every obese and overweight individual:

who is unaware of his/her obesity and its consequences.

who wants to lose weight but is not willing to change the present lifestyle.

who wants to change but from the next day, the next week, and so on.

who has changed the lifestyle and has started a program for it.

who had lost the weight but has regained it, perhaps more than before.

who is maintaining the lost weight.

who is experiencing and enjoying a healthy lifestyle.

– Sumedha

सर्वेंपि सुखिन सन्तु सर्वें सन्तु निरामया:।

सर्वें भद्राणि पश्यन्तु मा कश्चद् दु:ख माप्नुयात॥

LIFESTYLE MANAGEMENT TECHNIQUES FOR QUALITY LIFE

OBESITY AND EVERYTHING ABOUT IT

DR. SUMEDHA BHOSALE

notionpress.com

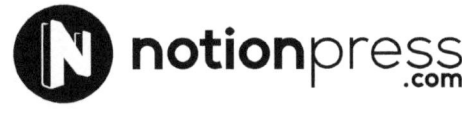

INDIA • SINGAPORE • MALAYSIA

Notion Press

Old No. 38, New No. 6
McNichols Road, Chetpet
Chennai - 600 031

First Published by Notion Press 2019
Copyright © Sumedha Bhosale 2019
All Rights Reserved.

ISBN 978-1-68466-724-6

Contents

Section I

Obesity

Section II

Psychology and Health Screening

Section III

Lifestyle Management through Healthy Lifestyle

Section IV

Medical Aspects of Obesity

Section V

Wellness

Foreword

Dr. H. V. Sardesai
MD (BOM) FRCPMRCP
FICA (USA) FACCP (USA)
FAIID (IND) FMACS (IND)

World Health Organization defines 'health' as not merely an absence of illness or a deformity but a positive state of wellbeing—physically, mentally and socially. Many of our ailments affect one of these three aspects of health. But obesity affects all the three aspects of our health. It is seen in all strata of society. It also affects younger people, even school-going children. The incidence of obesity is rising globally. A large number of other ailments stem from obesity. Therefore, obesity is now a prime health problem and its control is of utmost importance.

Like any other aliment, obesity is the result of genetic and environmental factors. Little can be done about our genetic predisposition to obesity. That leaves us with our lifestyle, which is a major area that needs to be looked into. Lifestyle includes our aahar (diet), vihar (rest and activity), vichar (thinking) and aachar (actions and exercises). In the past few years, considerable research has been done in all these fields. There has been an exponential growth in our understanding of the metabolic activities that influence our caloric balance. It is difficult for anyone to keep updating knowledge in all these fields.

Dr. Mrs. Sumedha Bhosale has done an excellent job in writing this book 'Obesity and Everything About It' for everyone. The book gives all information on the scientific aspects of energy metabolism. Dr. Bhosale has used simple language to express technical details. One doesn't encounter any technical jargon anywhere in the book. The information is up-to-date, scientific and precise. The book takes into account all aspects of management of obesity, namely diet, exercises, cultural aspects, habits, effects on health, and possible modes of treatment. Dr. Bhosale's comments have come from her rich experience and thorough expertise in this subject. Experts have added chapters in their respective fields of specialty to understand all the facets of the problem.

All in all, this is almost an encyclopedia on obesity. The book is well written, very informative and full of practical tips. Such a book must be possessed, read and put to use in practically in every family. This book has fulfilled the need for comprehensive knowledge on the subject in one place. I congratulate Dr. Mrs. Sumedha Sanjay Bhosale for this excellent book. I wish her all the best in her life to fulfill her mission to make our society healthy.

Dr. Sanjay Gupte

I have been a member of Status Health Club for the last 13 years.

Status Health Club is not just a gym or a slimming center. It is a medical gym and a wellness club. Along with members who are oriented toward general fitness, people suffering from various medical conditions (whom we call 'special population') exercise at the club, as part of their treatment.

Every year, Sanjay and Sumedha organize a great get-together to felicitate the 'successful achievers' who have found relief from their medical condition, lost weight or are doing well in their lifestyle management program. I have witnessed almost all the programs at the club and I have seen all the prize winners achieving higher fitness levels after obtaining relief from their medical conditions.

Sumedha is very keen to discuss the medical problems of her clients and the lifestyle modifications she prescribes in her program, with the expertise of a medical panel.

Status Health Club has a wellness clinic attached to it. It plans various activities for the promotion of health along with preventive and curative measures like PCOS clinic, menopause clinic, adolescent weight management clinic, neurobics program for fitness of the brain in a later age, relaxation center and so on, under the guidance of experts in the respective fields.

As a senior doctor, I always like to participate in the medical activities of Status Health Club. I feel that when people do not feel well, they approach the doctor; and it is the doctor's duty to approach people to take care of their wellness, when they are well.

This book by Sumedha is a part of her recent program on obesity elimination and social awareness. The name of the book 'Obesity and Everything About It' is self-explanatory.

The book gives plenty of information on ways to lower cholesterol; protective foods; sources of calcium, antioxidant vitamins and iron; stress management techniques; and prevention of obesity. These are extremely useful in the present-day scenario.

The concept of realistic weight and approaches to be avoided during weight reduction must be well learned by everybody who wants to lose weight.

I wish Sumedha the best success she deserves for this book as well as for her programs and personal life.

Dr. Lily Joshi
MD Medicine
Consultant physician

All over the world, the problem of obesity is increasing at an alarming rate. People of all ages and sexes are equally affected by it.

Though there is a plethora of literature available on the subject globally, a systematic and comprehensive study of the Indian scene had been lacking so far.

Finally, the wait is over. A complete treatise on obesity is now available to every reader. Authored by Dr. Sumedha Bhosale, a fitness consultant from Aamche Pune, this book titled *Obesity and Everything About It* does what it promises to do, that is give all the relevant information about this dreadful disorder.

The most striking features of this compilation are thoroughness, meticulous attention to detail, and a heartfelt desire to spread health awareness. From the definition of obesity and its etiology (causation) to its pathophysiology, complications, management and prevention, this book answers a whole lot of questions and gives a lot of additional information.

Obesity is discussed in all its aspects and perspectives. The book gives useful tips about cooking, shopping and eating behavior. It dwells on exercises, psychological makeup, coping skills and adoption of healthy habits. It gives a lot of data about the prevalence of obesity, which is spreading from the West to East in epidemic proportions. Various experts in the medical field have given their valuable inputs on medical and surgical management, making this book a rich compilation.

Thus, it is amply evident that *Obesity and Everything About It* will prove to be an excellent guide to adopting a healthy lifestyle and enhancing the quality of life.

Dr. Jagadish Hiremath
DM (Cardiology), DNB (Cardiology)
International cardiologist

This book by Dr. Sumedha Bhosale on obesity is a unique and proud addition to the book flora of Pune. It covers the topic of obesity extensively and exhaustively. It is a difficult task to give so much scientific material on this subject. Though the topic is common, the path is less traveled. The scientific crux of the book is worth appreciating and the language is remarkably simple for anybody to read and digest.

It will become a reference book in many libraries and it will help the masses at large be aware of the problems of obesity and ways to get over it or avoid it. My great compliments to Dr. Sumedha Bhosale for this endeavor.

Preface

It is comparatively easier to author a book than write the preface for the same.

Why did I decide to write this book *Obesity and Everything About It* in English and then translate it to Marathi?

I have been dealing with the obese population of Pune for the last 25 years. More than 25,000 thousand clients have been benefited from my 'lifestyle management with a healthy lifestyle' program.

When I started my first obesity clinic 25 years ago, 70% of my clients were in the age group of 25–30 years. The remaining 30% were below the age of 25 years. Recently, in the last two years, more than 50% of my clients have been below the age of 25 years. About 30% of them are school-going or college-going youngsters and 20% of them are newly-employed. The remaining 50% are above the age of 35 years and are suffering from other lifestyle-oriented medical conditions like hypertension, diabetes, heart disease and arthritis, along with obesity.

Isn't this a situation in which we need to evaluate and take concrete steps to change our present lifestyle?

Today, we are living an automatized life. Most of the activities that used to require strenuous physical exertion are getting accomplished by machines with a simple push of a button. Automobiles, elevators, escalators, intercoms, remote control and new-age gadgets are minimizing our efforts and movements.

Junk food and fast food, which are easily available in every nook and corner of every city, town and village, are replacing nutritious, low-calorie homemade food.

There is competition in every field, which is exposing each and every one to a tremendous amount of stress.

Lack of physical activity, consumption of junk food, competition, pollution and environment changes are some of the salient features of today's lifestyle. This lifestyle is in itself a threat to health. Obesity is one of the major consequences of a poor lifestyle. Obesity is a disease and the root cause of various life-threatening disorders.

Status Health Club is a medical gym and a wellness club. It is different from other gyms and slimming centers as we provide various health programs for the benefit of society, as our contribution towards your health, under the supervision of our medical panel.

We have to educate the maximum population about the exact treatment of obesity.

Obesity is a big problem but bigger and graver are the instant solutions for obesity. Lose weight without exercise, lose weight without going to the gym, lose 10 kg in 25 days, lose weight by eating supplements instead of a meal, use belts and lose tummy, have a walk while sleeping in bed! All these slogans seem attractive, but they do not provide scientific medical solutions.

As a result, even though you lose weight, you do not maintain your weight. You regain not just your lost weight but additional kilos too. More fats appear in place of the lost, useful fat-free mass. You regret being this new obese person, to a point where you actually prefer your old lesser obese self.

During the last 15 years, more than 25,000 Puneites have become members of Status Health Club and have experienced our various health programs. Out of them, more than 1,500 obese clients who were willing to lose weight have successfully completed the weight-loss program.

Actually, these members are the primary source of my success. They have endorsed my scientific approach. They have boosted my confidence. They have inspired me to study more and more. I have successfully completed many national and international academic courses to enhance my knowledge in this subject, so that my clients would be further benefited. The information provided in this book has references to the syllabus of such courses. I have liberally used the illustrations from various textbooks. I have modified the standards by Indianizing them.

All my members offer me the credit for their successful weight loss, with great love and respect. They follow my advice religiously and faithfully. All of them are my good friends. They share with me all their confidential private secrets. This helps me learn the psychological aspects of obesity. Many have fought and cried during their moments of despair. My members and my friends have shared their ups and downs, their tremendous tension and depression, and ultimately their joy at achieving success during this tough journey of weight loss. Now we are a healthy and fit family. My family grows by the day.

Through my 'trainers training' course, I have trained more than 400 trainers who are spreading our mantra of a healthy lifestyle in society through their slimming centers or by providing services in various health clubs and gyms.

My staff in Status are my health missionaries and the real sculptors of my success. They devote 15 hours every day to clients who come in for weight-loss programs. They teach them simple exercises, give lots of permutations and variations, make their exercise sessions enjoyable, take good care of their health and continuously motivate them to achieve their targeted goals. My staff members are major contributors in my success. How else could I have treated as many as 25,000 clients!?

I am extremely happy to hand over this book to you.

The important message one should follow during weight-loss and maintenance programs:

During a weight reduction program, always have a realistic weight in mind. Think about the achievable goal, which you can maintain for your lifetime.

In the pursuit of the ideal weight, do not punish yourself through starvation or extremely strenuous exercise.

Don't curse yourself for your obesity. Your physiology, metabolism, genetics, hormones, psychology and so many other factors are responsible for your misbehavior, i.e. your physical inactivity and overeating, which lead to obesity.

Do not be ashamed. Do not panic. Do not rush into unhealthy ways to lose your extra weight very fast. Don't be unhappy. Do not fall prey to the vicious circle of losing and gaining weight.

Accept yourself positively. Take medical advice and, if necessary, psychiatric help. Change your lifestyle. Commit yourself to a new and healthy lifestyle.

Even 10% of weight loss provides many health benefits. As the first step, avail yourself of these benefits, enjoy them and maintain the lost weight. Then try to lose further.

Gain health and enjoy life to its fullest potential.

I want you to start your weight-loss program scientifically and immediately.

With this information, you can easily achieve your 'dream weight.' In case of any problems, feel free to contact us in person, by snail mail, phone or email.

Wish you lots of success and the best of health!

Yours in health
Sumedha

Experts' Opinions

Dr. Anuradha Sowani

It is a well-written, well-researched book, covering all aspects of obesity. Dr. Sumedha's personal experience, expert technical knowledge and tremendous amount of effort come through very well.

Dr. Parag Biniwale and Dr. Vaishali Biniwale

This book on obesity by Dr. Sumedha Bhosale gives us comprehensive information about obesity and its consequences on general health and during special situations.

Dr. Ashish Babhulkar

Congratulations to Dr. Sumedha and Sanjay for their enthusiasm and zeal in the field of health and fitness. Appreciation should go to Dr. Sumedha for taking tremendous efforts to include topics as diverse as pregnancy and childhood obesity. She has left no stone unturned to make this book a 'must buy and read' book.

Dr. Sachin Tapasvi

This book is the first of its kind, discussing health, lifestyle and exercise. Dr. Sumedha Bhosale gives a very detailed and vivid description of what is a healthy lifestyle and how to achieve the same.

Dr. Sanjay Salunke, MS Surgery (gastroenterologist)

This is a unique book because it has a chapter on energy and metabolism, which brings out, in very simple language, the mechanisms that run the administration of our body.

Dr. Shrihari Dhorepatil

'Obesity and Everything About It' is a book that is much needed in today's changing lifestyle of over-indulgence. The author, Dr. Sumedha, has compiled all the aspects of obesity through her own experience of 20 years, along with the contemporaries in the field. This book gives complete guidance for a healthy lifestyle. It is a must-read, whether one is overweight or not!

Acknowledgments

No author can claim to be solely responsible for a book of this magnitude. There are several people I have to acknowledge for their assistance in writing this book.

First and foremost, my gratitude goes to all the doctors who have contributed their valuable thoughts in the form of detailed information of the diseases and their association with obesity, which I have incorporated in my book. Their inputs have given authenticity to the information I have provided. I am grateful to all of them.

Copy editing is the most important task in the process of publishing a book. It was capably handled by my friend Neeta Yadwad. She not only did a good job of editing but she also spent many hours translating medical and technical terms and complex concepts into a language that could be understood by everybody. She treated herself as a representative of readers and sought clarification on every concept till she understood it perfectly. Then she suggested simple and appropriate words to my thoughts, till both of us were satisfied. I am extremely grateful to her.

My special thanks to Rohini Attarde, who entered the data into my laptop at timings very convenient to me and odd to everyone. Her sincerity, affection and care while handling the script is creditable.

I cannot forget the contribution of my staff, who handled the health club in my absence and consulted me only for mobile counseling, during the crucial period of completion of this book.

The comments in this book from a panel of medical experts are extremely valuable and important. I thank the experts for taking time out from their busy schedules to read the book in detail and give a whole-hearted endorsement to the healthy lifestyle formula given in this book.

My special thanks to Dr. Sanjay Gupte, a paternal figure, who is ever-ready to answer my basic questions, support every new project of Status and guide me in every aspect, with a constantly smiling face. He is the person who encouraged me to write this book. He was kind enough to write a foreword for the book, complimenting Status and its staff with glowing words.

Thanks to Dr. Lily Joshi, our energetic counselor and regular exerciser at Status, who encouraged me to write this book.

This acknowledgment will not be complete without thanking Dr. Nishikant Shrotri, philosopher and guide in my life.

I do not have enough words to thank Dr. H.V. Sardesai, a doyen of lifestyle management techniques, for his enthusiastic appreciation and foreword for this book. All my efforts in writing this book were truly rewarded when I received his blessings and well wishes. It was very gracious on his part to encourage a novice author like me in my maiden attempt.

I am sincerely grateful to my clients, who are an inspiration for my work, without whom this book would not have come into existence.

Last but not the least, the understanding, appreciation, encouragement and patience shown by my son Ranjeet and my dear husband Sanjay during the tedious task of writing this book are beyond compare. I take this opportunity to tell them how grateful I am to them for all the things they have done for me.

Section I

Obesity

- **Definition**
- **Measurements**
- **Consequences**
- **Causes**
- **Energy metabolism**

Chapter 1

What Is Obesity?

Introduction

Let us know what the present status of our body composition is. What is the percentage of useful fat-free mass, such as muscles, bones and other organs, and what is our fat percentage?

An accurate assessment of body composition is an integral part of a comprehensive health screening.

When you want to know everything about obesity and wish to have a normal, recommended body weight and body composition, it is advisable to get your body composition assessed.

At the initial stage, height and weight charts can be referred to get a general idea about how much overweight you are. But the main shortcoming of these charts is that they do not give you an idea of relative body composition.

Excess body fat, and not weight, is associated with health risks and we are interested in minimizing the fat percentage during a weight-loss program.

Body composition assessment will help you lose weight and ultimately manage the lost weight. This chapter addresses the common methods of estimating body composition, including weight measurements, height-weight tables, anthropometric techniques, bio-electrical impedance, near infrared interactance (NIA). Sophisticated and highly accurate methods such as DEXA (dual energy X-ray and absorptiometry) are also discussed in the chapter.

This chapter will help you know your progress level and ensure that you are following the correct treatment to lose fat and confirm that you are not losing the useful fat-free mass.

Assessment of body composition will help you establish an appropriate and a realistic weight goal.

Get ready to know about the first important step i.e. assessment of body composition to follow a safe and scientific medical treatment for your obesity.

Know Your Body Weight and Fat Percentage

When our weight, according to the standard table, is 10% more, then it can be said that we are overweight. Being overweight is a stage in which the weight exceeds a certain standard weight, based on the height of a person.

Obesity is a condition of excessive fatness, either general or localized. It is possible to be obese at an existing weight within normal limits according to the standard table of height and weight, just like it is possible to be overweight. A sedentary person who does very less physical activity can have obesity even though his weight is normal according to the height-weight chart. Whereas an athlete or a coolie can be overweight even though he is not obese. Generally, being overweight or obese tends to be parallel with one other. With reference to the height-weight chart, being overweight means the body weight is more than 10% of the ideal weight.

If your body weight is more than 20% of your ideal weight, then you are OBESE.

Height-weight tables are the reference tables that most individuals use to assess the appropriateness of their weights. These tables do not provide information on relative body composition. Actually, body composition is more important as it is an integral part of comprehensive health screening and is recommended for individuals who are about to begin a weight-loss or exercise program. The evaluation of body composition provides the correct information on the body's structural components, i.e. muscles, fats and bones.

It is important to remember that height-weight charts provide only the initial reference point for assessment of the degree of being overweight. It is a general guide for a person to know the suitable weight. These charts are often based on statistics from insurance companies and they show desirable healthy weights in relation to the height.

Measuring Body Height and Weight

- An accurate balance beam or digital scale designed for commercial use provides the best measure of weight.

- The scale should be placed on a flat, hard surface and preferably kept at the same place.

- Use of the same scale will give the exact measure.

- The weight must be checked at the same time.

- Whenever you check the weight, wear the same clothes or clothes of similar weight.

- Stand still and distribute the body weight evenly.

- The scale needs to be calibrated frequently.

- Women on contraceptive pills, women who suffer from premenstrual syndrome with fluid retention a few days prior to the menstrual period and women of menopausal age show additional weight because of fluid retention influenced by hormonal behavior. Medical consultation is required in these cases.

Height is best measured using a wall-mounted stadiometer. Some commercial balance beam scales come with a metal sliding stadiometer.

Estimating Frame Size

The height-weight chart includes adjustment of frame size.

An individual's frame size can be assessed by measuring the breadth of an elbow. One has to flex the elbow at a 90-degree angle with the upper arm parallel to the floor. Measure the distance between the epicondyles i.e. inside and outside projections of elbow bone of the humerus (bone of upper arm) with broad-faced calipers. The frame size can be determined with the help of the height-weight tables.

Height and weight chart for men and women above age 25; small frame			
Height		Weight (kg)	
Cm	Feet	Men	Women
147	4.10"	—	42 – 44.5
149.5	4.11"	—	42.5 – 46
152	5"	—	43.5 – 47
154.5	5.1"	—	45 – 48.5
157	5.2"	50.5 – 54.5	46.5 – 50
159.5	5.3"	52 – 56	47.5 – 51
162	5.4"	53 – 57	49 – 52.5
164.5	5.5"	55 – 58	50.5 – 54
167	5.6"	57 – 60	52 – 56
169.5	5.7"	59 – 64	53.5 – 57.5
172	5.8"	62 – 67	55 – 59.5
174.5	5.9"	63 – 69	57 – 61
177	5.10"	65 – 70	58.5 – 63.5
179.5	5.11"	66 – 71	61 – 65
182	6.0"	67 – 72	63 – 67
184.5	6.1"	68 – 73	—
187	6.2"	69 – 74	—
189.5	6.3"	70 – 75	—
182	6.4"	74 – 77	—

Medium Frame

Height		Weight (kg)	
Cm	Feet	Men	Women
147	4.10"	—	43.5 – 48.5
149.5	4.11"	—	44.5 – 50
152	5"	—	46 – 51
154.5	5.1"	—	47 – 52.5
157	5.2"	52.5 – 57	48.5 – 54
159.5	5.3"	54 – 59	50 – 55
162	5.4"	56 – 60	51 – 57
164.5	5.5"	59 – 63	52.5 – 58.5
167	5.6"	61 – 65	54.5 – 61
169.5	5.7"	62 – 67	56 – 63
172	5.8"	63 – 68	58 – 65
174.5	5.9"	65 – 71	60 – 66.5
177	5. 10"	67 – 73	62 – 68.5
179.5	5.11"	69 – 75	63.5 – 70
182	6.0	70 – 77	65 – 72
184.5	6.1"	73 – 80	—
187	6.2"	75 – 83	—
189.5	6.3"	77 – 86	—
192	6.4"	78 – 87	—

Large Frame

Height		Weight (kg)	
Cm	Feet	Men	Women
147	4.10 ·	—	47 – 55
149.5	4. 11"	—	48 – 55
152	5"	—	49.5 – 56.5
154.5	5.1"	—	51 – 58
157	5.2"	57 – 63	52 – 59.5
159.5	5.3"	59 – 65	53.5 – 61
162	5.4"	61 – 67	55 – 63
164.5	5.5"	63 – 69	57 – 64.5
167	5.6"	66 – 72	57 – 64.5
169.5	5.7"	67 – 74	58.5 – 66
172	5.8 "	68 – 76	60 – 68

174.5	5.9"	70 – 77	62 – 70
177	5.10·	72 – 79	64 – 71.5
179.5	5.11"	73 – 81	67.5 – 76
182	6.0	75 – 82	69.5 – 78.5
. 184.5	6. 1"	76 – 84	—
187	6.2"	78 – 86	—
189.5	6.3"	80 – 88	—
192	6.4"	82 – 89	—

Medium Frame Determined By Elbow Width

Women		Men	
Height (feet)	Elbow width (cm)	Height (feet)	Elbow width (cm)
4.9" – 4.11"	5.7	5.1" – 5.3"	6.4 – 7
4.11" – 5.2"	5.4 – 6.4	5.4" – 5.6"	6.7 – 7.3
5.3" – 5.6"	5.7 – 6.7	5.7" – 5.10"	7.0 – 7.6
5.1" – 5.10"	6 – 7	5.11" – 6.2"	7.3 – 7.9
5.11" – 6.1"	6.4 – 7.3	6.3" – 6.4"	1.6 – 8.3

Body Mass Index (BMI)

Body mass index is the more preferred method for assessing body fat.

BMI accounts for differences in body composition by defining the level of adiposity (fatness) according to the relationship between weight and height, thus eliminating dependence on frame size.

$$BMI = \frac{\text{Weight in kilograms}}{\text{(square of Height in meter)}} \frac{kg}{\left[m^2\right]}$$

This index has the least correlation with body-height correlation with independent measures of body fatness for adults, including the elderly.

Obesity is categorized according to three grades.

Grade I	BMI	25 to 29.9
Grade II	BMI	30 to 39.9
Grade III	BMI	40

A general BMI of 27 or more indicates obesity, with an increased risk of developing health problems. BMI values increase with age.

As BMI uses total body weight and not the estimates of fat and lean body mass separately in the calculation, it does not discriminate between the obese and the athletes with a more muscled body type. Therefore, body composition assessments should ideally be used in conjunction with BMI. (An athlete's weight is more than the weight of a sedentary person's with more fat and a lean body. BMI may misguide in this case.)

More useful estimates of body composition are made by BMI.

Anthropometry

Measurement of circumference and skinfold is an easier and less expensive method of assessment of body composition. Anthropometric measures can also be used to assess body fat distribution i.e. central or peripheral, upper or lower circumference measures can be used to assess body composition with significantly overweight and obese people. The exact anatomical landmark should be carefully used.

A non-elastic cloth or fiberglass measurement tape must be used. The tape should be periodically calibrated against a meter stretch to ensure that it has not been stretched.

A long tape can be used to assess those who are significantly overweight. Individual indentation of the skin must be avoided by pulling the tape tight enough to keep it in position.

Estimating Body Fat from Circumference Measure

In women

Body density = 1.168297 − (0.002824 × abdomen in cm) + (0.00000122098 × abdomen cm) − (0.000733128 × hips cm) − (0.000510477 × height) − (0.00021616 × age)

In men

BF% (Body fat%) = 47.371817 + (0.57777791480 × abdomen) + (0.25189114 × hips) + (0.21366088 × iliac) − (0.35595404 × weight)

In women

BF% = 0.1107 (x1) − 0.17666 (x2) + 0.14354 (x3) + 51.0330

where   X1 = abdominal girth in cm

X2 = height in cm

X3 = weight in kg

Estimating Body Fat Distribution

Abdominal obesity is known to increase health risk. It is important to assess individual body fat distribution.

The most widely used technique is 'waist to hip circumference ratio WHR.' This is a fast and reliable assessment of fat distribution.

Measurement of waist I Measurement of hips

Risk degree	Men	Women
High risk	*WHR > 1*	*WHR > 81*
Moderately high risk	*WHR 0.90 – 1*	*WHR 0.81 – 0.85*
Lower risk	*WHR < 0.90*	*WHR < 0.80*

Obtaining Accurate Skinfold Measures

In this method, the skinfold measurements at particular sites are taken with the help of calipers.

The reliability of skinfold measures of body fat is not as high as other methods. This method requires other predicts i.e. weight, height, age and activity level. Formal training is required to use calipers properly.

The skinfold technique is based on two assumptions:

a) Thickness of the subcutaneous adipose tissue reflects the contact proposition of total body fat.

b) Selected site represents the average thickness of adipose tissue throughout the body.

Exact site location is also different.

Bio-Electric Impedance Analysis (BIA)

It is a relatively inexpensive, safe and portable method of assessing body composition.

BIA analyzers are often programmed with prediction equations to assess body composition. These equations vary with height, weight, sex and age with resistance.

In significantly overweight and underweight individuals, such equations may not be accurate.

Near Infrared Interactance (NIR)

NIA uses the principle of light absorption and reflection to estimate body fat with the help of near infrared spectroscopy. This technique provides the chemical composition of the body.

Gender-specific equations are required to be developed and cross validated.

This technique is also not very accurate in very underweight and overweight individuals.

Dual Energy X-ray Absorptiometry (DEXA)

It is a very popular method for assessing body composition. It assesses total bone mineral as well as regional estimates of bone, fat and lean tissues. It uses three component models to predict body fatness. It can be used to measure the body composition across the lifespan.

Using body composition results to determine a reasonable body weight.

Realistic Body Weight for Overweight Individuals

Individuals who have a lifetime history of obesity, a strong family history of obesity, or medical or other conditions that make weight management more difficult will be unlikely to maintain their 'ideal' weight for more than a short period of time.

For such populations, setting a realistic goal is extremely crucial.

One should set the primary goal of reducing body weight by 10%.

After this primary goal is achieved, it is easier to identify the next reasonable and achievable goal, taking into account how the individual has coped with lifestyle changes made so far.

Consider the lowest weight in the last 21 years and that should be the goal weight initially.

This helps provide positive changes in cholesterol, blood pressure and lipid profile. This encourages the individual to achieve the goal weight. Maintaining it is very important and it is a great challenge.

Thus, it is more important to set a realistic goal of being healthy and fit.

Many people are not happy with realistic goals. Our society covets lean, athletic and beautiful bodies. One glance at male and female models on popular magazine covers will tell you this. Film stars are idolized as role models and motivation for weight loss. Crash dieting, food restrictions and excessive exercises can lead to significant health problems and eating disorders.

Healthy eating habits for the entire lifespan and moderate and safe exercises, which improve fitness and give enjoyment, are the newly favored lifestyle practices. These will lead you toward good health.

You have to embrace a new lifestyle, which you will follow for life. You have to find out your realistic weight. You have to achieve and maintain the goal weight and enjoy life.

Unrealistic goals with punishing diet plans and exercise regimes will lead to serious and potentially life-threatening psychiatric disorders.

Chapter 2

Obesity Matters

Introduction

Yes, obesity matters! Not just cosmetically!

If you are obese, not only do you not look good but you also don't feel good. This is because obesity exposes a person to several health hazards, affecting all the systems of the body. In that sense, obesity is a multi-system disorder.

Obesity may lead to hypertension (elevated blood pressure), cardiovascular diseases CVD (less blood supply to the heart due to narrowing of arteries supplying blood to the heart), diabetes (increased blood sugar level), hyperlipidemia (increased total cholesterol, LDL, triglyceride) and osteoarthritis (swelling of joints due to wearing of joint components like cartilage and bone ends).

In the last two years, the more alarming news is that the increasing obesity rates in children are exposing them to diabetes type II (maturity onset diabetes), CVD and hypertension.

*The risks associated with obesity are briefly discussed in this chapter. In section IV of this book, renowned medical experts have written in detail the connection between obesity and these life-threatening disorders and the management of these disorders with weight reduction, lifestyle management and adopting a **healthy lifestyle**.*

Even if you are not suffering from any such conditions, your commitment to a healthy lifestyle will bring you a host of benefits. Scientific weight management will help you prevent health risks.

A healthy lifestyle provides a safe and sensible way to prevent risk factors, manages the serious health conditions, and helps you lead a healthy and quality life.

Obesity is associated with several health problems and medical problems.

- Increased risk of coronary artery disease

- Hypertension (increased blood pressure)

- Elevated total cholesterol

- Lower HDL cholesterol

- Stroke

- Type II diabetes

- Gout (type of arthritis where uric acid crystals are deposited in the joints)

- Cancer (breast and uterine in women; colon, rectal and prostate in men)

- Sleep apnea

- Arthritis

- Gallbladder disorder

- Potential social and psychological consequences

- Diaphoresis (excessive sweating)

- Fatigue

- Orthopnea (need to sit up to breathe)

- Digestive distress

- Menstrual abnormalities

- Infertility

- Other endocrinal disorders

- Sexual behavioral problems

- Surgical complications

- Shorter life span, which leads to premature deaths

Cardiovascular Disease (Diseases of Heart and Blood Vessels)

Coronary artery disease – The artery supplying oxygenated blood to the heart is known as coronary artery.

In an obese person, due to a high-fat diet and a sedentary lifestyle, there is plaque formation in the blood vessels. This progresses over time. The thrombus formation causes narrowing of the coronary arteries that supply blood to the heart. This is called atherosclerosis.

When blood supply to the heart is hampered, it causes chest pain or angina, which may lead to death of that part of the heart muscle. If the total supply to that part is stopped, then this condition is called myocardial infarction i.e. a heart attack.

Increased total cholesterol and obesity are the risk factors of heart disease (two out of total seven risk factors).

(Refer to the chapter on obesity and heart disease by Dr. Jagdish Hiremath.)

Hypertension

Obesity is also associated with high blood pressure. For every 10-kg increase in weight, there will be a 3-mm Hg rise in systolic blood pressure and a 2-mm Hg rise in diastolic blood pressure. Furthermore, the longer an individual is obese, the greater is the likelihood of developing hypertension.

Weight reduction is one of the effective ways to reduce and ultimately control elevated blood pressure.

Stroke

Atherosclerosis (narrowing of arteries due to plaque formation) due to thrombosis in the arteries that supply blood to the brain leads to loss of blood supply to that part of the brain. This leads to a stroke.

As body weight increases, the risk of stroke also increases. This risk is higher in obese people compared to those who are not obese.

Hypercholesterolemia (Dyslipidemia)

Obesity leads to elevation of total cholesterol and LDL cholesterol i.e. bad cholesterol. HDL cholesterol i.e. good cholesterol is lowered in overweight people. The elevated ratio of LDL to HDL has been related to most measures of body composition, including body fat percentage (BMI and WHR).

Weight loss and a low-fat diet have been found to dramatically improve lipid profile. Exercise improves the HDL level i.e. level of good cholesterol.

Diabetes

80% of type II diabetics are young obese. Overweight adults are nearly four times more likely to develop diabetes compared to age-matched, normal-weight people.

As the body fat increases, insulin does not act effectively on the cells to reduce blood glucose level. Weight loss improves glucose tolerance, decreases insulin resistance, and reduces raised blood sugar level (hyperglycemia).

(Refer to the chapter on obesity and diabetes by Dr. Lily Joshi.)

Gallbladder Disease

Bile in gallbladder can become super saturated with cholesterol. In obese people, the motility of the gallbladder is reduced. This results in less efficient emptying. The next effect is an increased risk of gallstone formation in obese individuals. (Fat, fertile and flatulent females of 50 years tend to have a higher incidence of gallstones.)

Respiratory Diseases

In obese people, the respiratory function is frequently impaired. Increased fat in the chest decreases the mechanical efficiency of the respiratory system. Excess fats in the viscera may compromise the efficient motion of the diaphragm and the rib cage. The total lung capacity tends to be lower. Fatty tissue may obstruct the large airways, leading to sleep apnea and orthopnea (i.e. need to sit up to breathe) in many cases.

Arthritis

Stress on weight-bearing joints increases as weight increases. This often leads to arthritis. Knee, hip and lower back problems are frequently reported by obese people. Excessive wearing of knee and hips joints can lead to degeneration of these joints, particularly as the severity and duration of obesity increase.

(Refer to the chapter on obesity and knee joints by Dr. Sachin Tapasvi.)

Health-related quality of life is dramatically affected as mobility and simple daily tasks are much more difficult for obese people.

The health-related effects on quality of life due to obesity are:

- Increased shortness of breath

- Decreased mobility and range of movement

- Diminished capacity of exercise and activity

- Increased ankle swelling

- Lower level of physical self-efficacy i.e. perception of one's ability to exercise

- Decrease agility and balance

- Backache (Refer to the chapter on obesity and osteoarthritis and backache by Dr. Ashish Babhulkar.)

- General fatigue

Digestive Distresses

Along with gallstone formation, the liver too is adversely affected. Degenerative diseases of liver and cirrhosis of liver strike obese person more often. Some diseases of the colon (di-ventricular disease of colons) and piles are associated with obesity.

Gynecological Disorders

Irregular menstruation, polycystic ovarian diseases and infertility are common in obese women and vice versa i.e. these disorders lead to obesity. A vicious circle sets in; it can be broken by weight reduction. (Refer to the chapter on obesity and PCOS by Dr. Sanjay Gupte.)

Obesity creates many problems during pregnancy. Generally, obese women do not experience normal delivery.

(Refer to the chapter on obesity and pregnancy by Dr. Parag Biniwale and Dr. Vaishali Biniwale.)

Endocrinal System

Several endocrinal functions and obesity are closely associated with each other and they are interdependent. Many times, disfunction of one hormone disturbs the function of every gland and the total physiology.

Excessive Sweating

Fat people perspire profusely as they have to spend a lot of energy to do any physical work. Layers of fat act as woolen jackets or sweaters and cause profuse perspiration, which emits a foul odor, causing great embarrassment to the person.

Obesity and Cancer

The risk of cancer is 10% greater among obese people. Compared to other women, overweight women are more prone to cancers of the breast, esophagus (food pipe) and reproductive organs in general and the uterus in particular.

40% of overweight men are more prone to cancers of the intestine and prostate.

(Refer to the chapter on obesity and cancer by Dr. Anuradha Sowani.)

Potential Psychological and Social Problems

Obese people commonly suffer from lack of confidence, inferiority complex, low self-esteem and depression.

Gossip, taunts, ridicule and difficulty in getting clothes, a life partner or a suitable job are some of the social problems that obese people face, leading to psychological disorders.

Sexual Problems

Many times, obesity leads to sexual problems. The blood vessels supplying blood to sexual organs, like the coronary arteries, get narrowed because of atherosclerosis. Partial impotency may be the consequence of this. Lack of confidence and low self-esteem may worsen the problems. Weight reduction through exercise helps a lot in this situation, as the testosterone secretion is stimulated with resistance training. The resultant improvement in sexual performance helps resolve other psychological disorders like depression.

Obesity and Surgery

A lot of contemplation is required on the part of the surgeon before performing surgery.

It is very difficult to locate the body part hidden under a mass of fat and then perform surgery. It is also dangerous for an anesthetist to administer anesthesia to an obese person. The breathing of an overweight person is shallow, as the movement of his diaphragm is hindered. Anesthesia is likely to affect his breathing adversely. There are chances of developing embolism in the veins. Moreover, post-surgical recovery is very slow in an overweight person. The convalescence period is also usually very long.

Surgical operations in the treatment of gallstones, appendicitis, piles, hernia, cancer of the intestine, prostate, and varicose veins are difficult to perform in obese people. Consequently, the individuals are deprived of proper treatment.

Obesity and Life Expectancy

Extensive research indicates that obesity is a major factor in reducing life expectancy. Diseases caused by obesity lead to untimely demise.

Chapter 3

Energy Formation and Metabolism

Introduction

This chapter presents information about energy metabolism in detail. The factors responsible for energy expenditure, such as resting metabolism rate, thermic effect of food and thermic effect of exercise, provide information about the reasons for obesity.

The information about the structure of fat cells, fat depots, fat distribution, fat cell development, sources of lipids in fat cells and role of enzymes in the regulation of fat percentage tell us why some people are obese, even though they do not overeat. With this information, we can understand that obesity is a complex phenomenon and several factors are responsible for this condition. It is not just improper eating habits like overeating and lack of physical activity that lead to obesity but many other factors are involved in the phenomenon.

The chapter presents information in the form of medical and technical terminology. Knowing it will help you choose the scientifically correct treatment for weight reduction.

The balance between energy expenditure and energy intake ultimately determines whether an individual will lose or gain weight.

When you decide to lose weight, try to understand the factors that influence energy balance.

It is very simple to understand this. If energy intake is more than energy output, weight gain occurs. This is a positive energy balance. If energy expenditure is greater than energy intake, weight loss occurs. This is a negative energy balance. When energy intake is equal to energy expenditure, the weight is maintained.

Even though this concept is very simple to understand, human physiology is very complicated. It involves many factors.

Energy balance is a simple relationship between the number of calories consumed by you and all the calories expended by you—for just being alive and awake i.e. resting metabolic rate plus all the calories required to perform your daily physiological and physical work. This includes the energy required for activities like sitting, getting up, walking and climbing stairs.

This resting metabolic rate (RMR), which includes basal metabolic rate (BMR), is about 60–75% of the daily energy expenditure. Even though you are not doing any physical activity, your body is continuously performing many tasks like cardiac function (keeping your heart beating), neural function (function of the nerves) and repair of body cell and structure, even in the absence of physical activity. RMR is directly related to fat-free mass, as all the activities of life are conducted by fat-free mass alone. Greater the fat-free mass, higher is the RMR. The most commonly used measurement is RMR (than BMR). BMR is approximately 10% lower than RMR. RMR in women is at least 1200 kcal/day and in men it is 1500 kcal/day. In many cases, the values are higher than these.

The costs of digestive processes (thermic effect of food) are about 10% of the daily energy expenditure.

Proteins require more energy to get broken down into amino acids. Complex carbohydrates also require more energy to get converted into sugar after digestion. Large fat molecules require comparatively less energy than proteins and complex carbohydrates.

The cost of activity (thermic effect of activity) is responsible for about 15–30% of the total daily energy output. Obviously, if the physical activity is increased, the energy expenditure also gets increased. In a sedentary person (who does less physical activity), only 15% of the total daily energy expenditure comes from his activities. Whereas if a person is highly active, this number jumps to 30% or more. Even though many factors affect energy expenditure, 'physical activity' is the best way to increase your calorie expenditure.

Energy Production during Physical Activity

The energy we require to do work comes from food. The food we eat gets digested; the carbohydrates get converted into sugar, proteins get converted into amino acids and fats get converted into fatty acids. The primary function of carbohydrates and fats is to provide energy. When enough carbohydrates are not consumed, proteins have to provide energy.

Muscles contract and exert force. The energy used to drive the contraction comes from adenosine triphosphate. The glucose is broken down to provide adenosine triphosphate i.e. ATP. How quickly and efficiently a muscle cell produces ATP determines how much work the cell can do before it gets fatigued. Some ATP is already stored in some muscle cells. For muscle contraction (forced) to happen, stored ATP and newly produced ATP get utilized. If we want to continue this work, muscle cells have to produce ATP continuously. This production of ATP takes place in three ways.

- Aerobic system

- Anaerobic energy system

- Anaerobic creatinine phosphate system

Aerobic energy system: Aerobic means 'in the presence of oxygen.' In aerobic exercises like running, hill climbing and aerobic dance workout, the heartbeat is increased on purpose to supply more oxygen to the cells to meet energy production needs. Even when the muscle cells are at rest, more oxygen is delivered to the cells. Each cell, even the muscle cell, contains structures called mitochondria. They can be called 'power stations' as they are the sites where aerobic energy (ATP) is produced. The greater the number of mitochondria, the greater is the cell's capacity to produce energy.

When the aerobic activity is continued, energy is produced from fats.

Anaerobic energy system: When a muscle needs to generate force quickly, such as when a person lifts a heavy weight, during gym or resistance exercises, in the absence of additional oxygen, the muscle provides a rapidly available source of ATP. This ATP is produced from glycogen stores in the muscles. When predominantly heavy muscle movements, like running or cycling are performed, at an intensity greater than an individual's functional aerobic capacity, then ATP production happens anaerobically. This anaerobic production occurs in the cell, outside the mitochondria. Characteristically, lactic acid is produced, which causes temporary fatigue or a burning sensation after the creation of large force by muscle cells.

It is important to know that there is continuous energy production, either through the aerobic or anaerobic system. Energy production does not work like an on/off switch. It is a matter of predominance. When adequate oxygen is not available in the mitochondria of a cell to meet ATP needs, the anaerobic system kicks into high gear to assist the aerobic system. The anaerobic system does not shut off.

Most cells, such as the cells of the heart, brain and other organs, have very little or no anaerobic capability. These cells require a continuous supply of oxygen. Blockage of the artery into the brain can lead to a stroke. Whereas skeletal muscles have significant anaerobic capability. Fatty acids from fats and glucose from carbohydrates are the two sub-straits used to produce most of the ATP supply.

Proteins are not preferred energy sources. In case you do not produce energy through aerobic system, the primary source of ATP production is fatty acids and glucose. The byproducts of aerobic ATP production are water and carbon dioxide. The body eliminates both these byproducts easily and you do not get rapid muscle fatigue.

It is extremely important to note that when energy is produced through the aerobic system, water is a byproduct. Every day, we lose a lot of water in order to regulate our internal temperature. Both aerobic and anaerobic systems produce heat. This heat is transported to the skin. From the skin, the heat is dissipated into the environment in the form of sweat. Even during rest, there is continuous aerobic energy production, as we discussed earlier. As the energy production is at a low rate, the water produced is evaporated before reaching the skin's surface. This is insensible perspiration.

When the intensity of exercise increases, heat production increases. Water loss also increases. As the duration of exercise increases, then obviously the loss of water from the body increases.

Take into consideration this increased loss of water, along with regular water loss throughout the day. It is extremely important that you drink enough water throughout the day. At least eight to ten glasses of water are required by a person who does normal day-to-day routine. You have to add a minimum of two glasses of water for one hour of physical exercise of moderate intensity.

Adequate hydration is necessary for maintaining fluid balance. Inadequate water intake can lead to a water retention problem. In addition to temperature regulation, adequate hydration is important to replenish the glycogen stores in muscle cells, as each gram of glycogen is stored along with 4 grams of water.

An overweight person needs more water than a slim person. Additionally, water helps in maintaining proper muscle tone. Without adequate hydration, the blood supply to the working muscle may not be able to provide adequate oxygen to perform exercises, which leads to unbearable muscle cramps and sometimes joint pain. Drinking water helps keep the blood pumped up with oxygen. It is necessary to lubricate the joints and provide a cushion to organs and tissues. Inadequate water intake leads to sunken eyes, dark circles and dull, dry skin, as fluid drains and the skin gets bruised.

Digestion and excretion of waste require adequate water intake. High-fiber food does not get digested when there is lack of water and the food gets cemented to the intestines. With adequate water intake, the flow of digestive juices is also adequate.

Inadequate water intake leads to dryness of the mouth and furry tongue and prevents bacteria on teeth from being washed away, resulting in bad breath (halitosis). Absorption and transportation of nutrients require enough water intake.

If your diet does not provide sufficient carbohydrates for energy production, then the body is capable of using protein that is stored in tissues like muscles to produce the energy it needs. This process is known as gluconeogenesis. This occurs to a limited extent, but it is not healthy to rely on it for substantial energy production.

Gluconeogenesis, combined with abnormal fat metabolism results in ketosis, where the levels of blood acids are increased.

In the presence of adequate oxygen in the mitochondria of cells, ATP is produced from fatty acids and glucose. This suggests that, during rest, the mitochondria produces most of the ATP needed, in the presence of oxygen from fatty acids and glucose.

When oxygen use increases, calorie expenditure also increases. For one liter of oxygen used, approximately five kilocalories of energy are utilized. Intensity of exercise, amount of oxygen utilized and calorie expenditure are dependent on each other.

The body utilizes about 1 to 1.5 kcal per minute at rest. Actually, this expenditure is related to a number of factors. Fat-free mass, i.e. lean body mass, is a significant component, which decides actual energy expenditure.

About 50–60% of this 1-to-1.5-kcal-per-minute energy is derived from fatty acids in a normal person. Whereas in well-trained endurance athletes, fatty acids provide 70% of resting calorie expenditure.

There are many myths surrounding the energy expenditures. Some of them are:

- One utilizes muscle sugar supply before fat can be used.

- It takes 20 minutes of exercise before fat begins to be used for energy production.

Actually, fat is used for energy production even during sleep, although in very a less percentage.

As exercise intensity increases, the cardiovascular system responds in the following manner to the increased intensity:

- Heart rate is increased.

- Stroke volume is increased.

- Oxygen extraction in the active muscle fibers increases, so that delivery of oxygen to the mitochondria of exercising muscle improves. Aerobically more ATP is produced.

As long as sufficient oxygen is available, continuously more and more ATP is produced. The aerobic system predominates and calorie expenditure per minute increases substantially above the resting rate.

At some point during the increasing intensity, there is not enough oxygen available in the mitochondria of the exercising muscle to meet the energy needs. This point is determined by genetics and your level of fitness. At this point, the anaerobic systems are called upon to rapidly produce ATP. This stage of intensity at which adequate oxygen is not available is typically referred to as 'lactate threshold' or 'anaerobic threshold.' At an intensity above the threshold, the aerobic system does not stop working; but it cannot produce enough ATP to meet the energy demands at that pace. Here, anaerobic systems provide the necessary energy, above and beyond the aerobic capability.

At maximum effort, anaerobic systems work at maximum capability. The primary source of the anaerobic system of ATP production is glucose. Carbohydrates after digestion get converted into glucose. Glucose is carried in the blood and stored in the liver and muscle cells as glycogen. Glycogen is a large molecule made up of chains of glucose. From glycogen, an individual glucose molecule is broken down to enter the energy pathway. If you understand how the energy is utilized, this knowledge will help you make a better food choice, which will replenish your body for its particular needs.

Losing Body Fat

Fat store is the primary energy reserve of a well-nourished body. This fat is stored as triglycerides in the adipose cells around the body as well as in the skeletal muscle fibers. Carbohydrate stores in the form of glycogen are relatively less and protein is not a preferred source of energy. With this knowledge, you can understand how the energy balance is related to body fat. One 1 kg of fat is equal to 7,600 kilocalories. We have to understand that we need to burn 7,600 kcal more to lose 1 kg of fat. In other words, we have to create a negative balance of 7,600 kcal, for 1-kg weight loss (in ten days.)

Creating negative energy balance is best accomplished by increasing calorie expenditure and moderately reducing the calorie intake.

The key to maximizing fat loss is to maximize calorie expenditure. If you are untrained and can do exercises with an intensity of about 5 kcal/min, then during a onehour session of exercise, you will burn a minimum of 300 kcal per session per day. And when you will eliminate about 400 to 500 kcal/day, then in a month you will create a negative energy balance of 24,000 kcal. This means you will lose 3.5 kg weight in a month.

Even when your level of fitness is dramatically improved, three to four months after beginning a training program, your exercise intensity may reach 12 kcal/min. This will lead to 600 kcal/day for 50 minutes of workout. Even if you exercise four times a week, you can easily lose half kg of weight per week, by restricting your calorie intake to 400 to 500 kcal per day, along with exercise.

When you exercise aerobically, you are able to use more fat for ATP production at any intensity. This helps the body spare the muscle store of glycogen.

Fat burns in the flame of glucose. Glucose releases pyruvic acid after breaking down. From pyruvic acid, ATP production takes place in the mitochondria. The fat can enter the process of energy production only if enough pyruvic acid is present along with oxygen.

Improved aerobic fitness enhances the capacity to use stored fat for ATP production. Even though you are untrained, you can understand that aerobic exercise is essential for you, as it can sustain long enough to burn significant calories. Anaerobic exercise helps improve lean body mass, which is responsible for increased demand of calories during exercise and for metabolic demands.

The additional energy expenditure is due to the increased AMR after a bout of exercise.

During recovery phase, oxygen requirement increases. This is referred to as excess post-exercise oxygen consumption (EOPC). The oxygen need is referred to as oxygen debt. Oxygen debt includes oxygen deficit, accumulated at the outset of a bout of exercise, plus oxygen required for recovery of respiratory muscle-elevated enzyme activity and reloading of oxygen on myoglobin molecule.

The intensity and duration of exercise has the most significant impact on EOPC. Aerobic exercise increases the post-exercise metabolic rate up to 17–24 hours. Heavy resistance training may lead to even longer increase in EPOC.

It is difficult to understand the complicated biochemical pathways. This is the simplified and brief description of energy production. It will make you understand that if you want to maximize fat metabolism, you have to exercise with moderate intensity for a longer duration. This ensures calorie expenditure increases to achieve weight loss through utilization of maximum fat.

Even though theoretically we calculate and expect a certain amount of calorie expenditure for certain types of exercise, the expected weight loss and actual results depend on so many other factors like your age, gender, activity level and genetics. Many other factors also affect the weight loss. They include the set point theory. Simultaneously, during weight loss, there is some unavoidable lean body loss, which causes the loss of AMR. Both losses attenuate the overall impact of calorie expenditure.

The Fat Depot (Development, Store, Regulation and Factors Responsible for Fat Deposition)

The balance between energy expenditure and energy intake keeps your body weight constant. The complex system of neural, hormonal and chemical mechanisms is responsible for this energy balance. Abnormalities in any of the mechanisms are responsible for weight abnormalities. All the mechanisms have still not been understood completely.

We have learned that a body weight 20% above the desirable weight means obesity and 40% above the desirable weight means severely obesity. We have to understand that obesity is a more complex issue than a matter of self-control. Overeating and lack of physical activity are not the only reasons of obesity. Physiologic, metabolic and genetic factors are also responsible for an undesirable physical state.

Components of Body Weight

Let us look at the components of body weight. Body weight is the sum of bones, muscles, organs, body fluids and adipose tissue. All these components keep on changing their size and weight during various phases in life, like growth, reproductive stage, variation in exercise level and aging. About 60% of our body weight is due to water. The state of hydration can fluctuate the weight across several kilos. The adipose tissue keeps on changing due to several mechanisms discussed earlier. As this tissue increases in weight, bones and muscles support its burden to some extent. However, most of the gain in fats causes the change in the size of the fat depots beneath the skin. Tissue or body components other than fat are known as lean body mass (LBM). It is higher in men and lower in women and elderly.

Let us learn more about the adipose tissues.

Fat is the primary energy reserve of the body. It is stored as triglycerides in depots made up of adipose tissue. In women, the appropriate body fatness ranges from 20–25% of the total body weight. Out of this, 12% is essential fat. Essential fat includes an extra 5–9% sex-specific body fat in the breasts, pelvic region and thighs. In men, the appropriate body fatness is 12–15% of the body weight. Out of that, 4–7% is essential fat. This essential fat in both sexes includes fat stored in the bone marrow, heart, lung, liver, spleen, kidneys, intestines, muscles and lipid-rich tissues in the nervous system. It is necessary for normal physiological functioning. Storage fat is the fat that accumulates in the adipose tissues under the skin and around internal organs to protect them from trauma. The totality of fat stores in the adipocyte (fat cell) is capable of extensive variation.

Structure

Adipose tissue is located primarily under the skin in the mesenteries and omentum and behind the peritoneum (inner structures of the abdomen).

It is of two types: white adipose tissue and brown adipose tissue. White adipose tissue serves as a repository for triglycerides and forms a cushion to protect abdominal organs. It also acts as an insulator to preserve body heat. It looks slightly yellowish due to the presence of carotene.

Brown adipose tissue is seen in infants and in very small amounts in adults. It occurs primarily in the scapular (bones at the back) and sub-scapular areas. The brown color is due to extensive vascularization (network of blood vessels).

Regional Distribution

Four types of obesity are recognized. They are:

- Excess body mass or percentage fat

- Excess subcutaneous (under the skin) truncal abdominal fat (android)

- Excess abdominal visceral fat

- Excess gluteo-femoral fat (gynoid)

Regional patterns of fat deposits are controlled genetically. They differ between and among men and women. The gynoid type is more common in women. This is characterized by a pear shape that is created by heavier deposits of fat around the thighs and buttocks. These deposits are presumed as energy reserves to support the demands of pregnancy and lactation.

The android or apple shape is more common among men. It is characterized by the presence of fats around the waist and upper abdomen. Free fatty acids from the fats depots are mobilized rapidly. This type of obesity is associated with significant risk for hypertension, cardiovascular disease, maturity onset or non-insulin dependent diabetes mellitus. Many times in women, there is a combination of both gynoid and android type obesity.

Adipocyte

The mature adipocyte consists of large central lipid droplets surrounded by a thin rim of cytoplasm. It contains the nucleus and mitochondria. Adipocytes store fat in quantities equal to 80–95% of their volume.

Hypertrophy and Hyperplasia

Hypertrophy means increase in size. Hyperplasia means increase in the number of fat cells.

Weight gain may be the result of hypertrophy or hyperplasia of adipocytes or a combination of both. Obesity is always characterized by hypertrophy; only some forms of obesity also involve hyperplasia. The fat depots can expand as much as 1,000 times through hypertrophy alone. Hypertrophy is a process that can occur any time as long as space is available in the adipocytes. Hyperplasia occurs as part of the growth process, during infancy, adolescence, and sometimes even in adulthood (when the fat content of the cells reaches the upper limit of the cells' capacity). When weight is reduced because of starvation, illness, trauma or changes in diet and exercise, the size of fat cells decreases.

Hyperplasia, i.e. increase in the number of cells, can take place at any stage of life. When the cell reaches its maximum size, i.e. when there is full hypertrophy, hyperplasia takes place. With weight loss, the size of the cell reduces but the number of cells does not. Prevention is the only answer because once the fat is gained and maintained over time it may become permanent. After weight loss, the reduced or half empty fat cells are unhappy and hungry and seek to restore normal volume. Weight loss is more difficult to achieve and weight is regained more easily in hypercellular obesity than in obesity of the hypertrophic kind.

Development of Fat Cells

At the age of six months, the greatest level of fatness in normal growth occurs. In lean children, the size of the fat cell decreases. In obese children, it does not decrease. In normal children, there is a gradual increase in fatness again at the age of six years. In girls, this increase is greater than in the boys. The cell number increases in both lean and obese children, throughout childhood up to adolescence, but the number increases faster in obese children than in lean children. After adolescence, hypertrophy occurs primarily. The gradual increase of fats in obese children starts even before they reach the age of five years.

Storage of Fat

The fat in adipose tissue comes directly from dietary fats. Excess carbohydrates and proteins are converted into fats, but this process is comparatively slower. Even though 1 gm of fat provides 9 kcal, dietary fat provides more than 9 kcal (up to 11 kcal) energy, which can be metabolized. Conversion of carbohydrates into fats requires additional energy, which is three times than that of fats. This suggests that we have to consider the total amount of calories we are consuming as well as restrict the percentage of calories from fats.

Even though diet composition is important, it is not just an issue of fats. Total calories are also important. So, you eat low-fat food but you don't forget the calories. If you have to lose weight, control fat and also consume food with low calories.

Action of Lipoprotein-Lipase Enzyme

The fats we eat get converted into triglycerides during digestion. Triglyceride is transported to the liver as part of chylomicrons and is removed from the blood by the enzyme lipoprotein lipase. Lipoprotein lipase is present at the end part of the capillaries (smallest blood vessels). This enzyme is responsible for the entry of lipids into the adipose cells from the blood through the walls of the capillaries.

Triglyceride is synthesized in the liver from fatty acids. Triglyceride gets attached to very-low-density lipoprotein particles (VLDL). It is transported to the cells. At the periphery of the blood vessel, it gets removed from the blood by lipoprotein lipase (LPL). This enzyme causes hydrolysis of triglycerides into free fatty acids and glycerol. The glycerol proceeds to the liver and the fatty acids enter the adipocyte. In adipocytes, the fatty acids are reconverted into triglycerides. If they are required by other cells to produce energy, once again they are converted into fatty acids and glycerol through the action of hormone-sensitive lipase (HSL). Fatty acids and glycerol reconverted through this phenomenon re-enter the blood vessels.

Hormones affect LPL activity in different adipose tissue regions. In the gluteo-femoral region, estrogen stimulates LPL activity. Due to this, storage of fat is promoted in this area. However, in the abdominal area, estrogen stimulates lipolysis. After menopause, due to lack of estrogen, there is a marked fat deposition around the abdomen.

During the weight gain period, LPL increases in both obese and non-obese people. After weight loss, LPL returns to a normal level in non-obese people. Whereas in obese people, the LPL does not decrease. In fact, it increases. This is a major factor for rapid weight regain. LPL is also higher in smokers. This leads to weight gain after they quit smoking. In genetically obese people, the levels of LPL are characteristically high.

Mechanism of Regulation of Body Weight

A variety of regulatory systems exist in our body to maintain weight at some predetermined point. When you eat food, the catecholamines, nor-epinephrine and dopamine are released by the sympathetic nervous system (SNS). These are neuro transmitters. They are responsible for the feeding behavior of the hypothalamus, which is the part of the brain that controls hunger. Fasting and semi starvation lead to decreased SNS activity and increased adrenal medullary activity. Due to this, there is an increase in epinephrine, which fosters mobilization.

Short-Term and Long-Term Regulation of Body Weight

Regulation of body weight takes place on a short-term and long-term basis. Short-term regulation governs the consumption of food from meal to meal. Long-term regulation is controlled by the availability of adipose tissue.

Short-term regulation

Short-term controls are primarily related to hunger, appetite and satiety. Satiety is associated with the state after a meal, when excess food is being stored. Hunger is associated with the state after absorption of food when the stores after meal are mobilized. In old age, spontaneous short-term changes cannot be controlled. Appetite (desire for food) is usually triggered by the thought of food or food itself.

Long-term regulation

When normal body composition is disturbed during weight loss because of any reason, signals are sent from the adipose tissues and a feedback mechanism is activated. This mechanism is prominently observed in younger people. The requirement of fats for energy production is fulfilled by the adipose tissue.

Set Point Theory

Fat storage in non-obese adults is regulated and specific body weight is preserved. When we try to lose weight by starvation, the body rapidly returns to the original weight as if the original weight was taken as 'a set point' constituted by the body. This set point is suitable and amenable to physiological influences. This theory tells us that any abnormality established in the set point is the reason for some type of obesity.

The body weight remains remarkably stable in spite of variations. This may be because of a genetically-determined internal regulatory mechanism. If the weight is at its normal level, then only metabolism is normal. There is a 5%-drop in weight, which results in a 15%-drop in resting metabolism. This drop is for an effort to regain the weight that is lost. The body makes a series of internal adjustments to resist weight change and conserve fat stores through an internal control-mechanism, which is probably located in the hypothalamus.

Recent study says that if newly lost weight is maintained over a long time, then the set point adjusts to a new level. But overeating, lack of exercise, lesions in the brain and drugs may disturb the new set point. Dieting is generally futile, unless the set point is lowered by maintaining a lowered weight.

Plateau Effect

An important aspect of the set point theory is that a plateau in weight loss is common. In spite of regular exercise and proper calorie control, the weight does not get lowered for many days. If calorie control is maintained, additional weight loss should occur. This generally happens for the last few kilos that have to be lost, before the ideal healthy body weight is reached.

During a weight reduction program, the weight remains at the same level for a period of time. Weight loss halts completely. The lipid level in the adipose tissues reduces to some point. This demands metabolic adjustment and weight maintenance.

With weight loss, LBM is lost, which results in the rapid dropping of RMR. This drop is to adapt to the new low weight and face deprivation.

Reduced food intake leads to reduced thermic effect of food. Body with less weight requires less energy expenditure to move around, so that the cost of physical activity is also less. A state of equilibrium is reached eventually. At this stage, energy intake is equal to energy expenditure.

At this stage, either a change in diet or in physical activity is required, so that there is further weight till the next plateau is reached.

Thermo Genesis and Thermogenic Effect of Food (TEF)

In the first part of this chapter, we discussed the components of energy expenditure. They are:

- resting energy expenditure (REE), expressed as RMR

- energy expended in physical activity

- thermogenic effect of food or diet-induced thermo genesis

Obligatory thermo genesis is energy required for digestion, absorption and metabolizing nutrients. The metabolic rate is increased by 5% after consumption of carbohydrates and fats. It increases by 25% after consumption of proteins and increases by 10% when a liberal mixed diet is consumed.

Adaptive thermo genesis is an increase in metabolic rate stimulated by eating, followed by exercises, when TEF almost doubles. Cold, caffeine and cigarette also stimulate TEF. Diet-induced thermo genesis is higher after breakfast and declines as the day progresses.

Resting Metabolic Rate

Starvation or semi starvation results in a dropping of RMR by 15% in two weeks. It returns to normal when adequate food intake is restored.

Gut Peptides

Gut peptides like cholecystokinin get secreted when the mucosa of stomach and small intestine get stimulated after fullness because of mechanical contact with food. They have an immediate effect on satiety. You get a feeling of fullness and tend to stop eating. Some of the gut peptides are also found in the brain where they stimulate and inhibit eating.

Brain Proteins

Galatin, the natural brain protein, rises throughout the morning. It stimulates an appetite for fats at lunch. It continues to rise till dinner.

This protein is higher in adolescent girls. This may be the provision for pregnancy. Some neuro proteins cut fat intake. There is ongoing research to find a medication to control appetite without disrupting other bodily functions.

Thyroid Hormones

Adaptive thermo genesis discussed earlier (increase in metabolic rate due to exercise) improves because of thyroid hormones. Tissue responsiveness to the catecholamines secreted by the central nervous system is increased.

The decrease in T3 causes diminished adaptive thermo genesis. This is the factor that causes excessive weight gain in a person with hypothyroidism (a condition where thyroid hormones secretion is subnormal).

Insulin

Increased level of insulin leads to increase in food intake. Insulin causes a decrease in the sugar level i.e. hypoglycemia. As sugar lowers, one gets stimulated to eat. If insulin level is impaired, SNS activity is reduced and this leads to reduced thermo genesis. Obese people with insulin resistance or insulin deficiency have a defective glucose disposal system and a depressed level of thermo genesis.

Fasting insulin levels increase in obese people. However, many obese individuals show insulin resistance, less glucose tolerance and increased cholesterol levels (hyper lipidemia). This sequence gets corrected if weight is lost, through diet control and exercise.

Chapter 4

Nature and Causes of Obesity

Introduction

We learned about metabolism and energy production in our body in detail. This helped us understand the complex phenomenon of obesity.

The imbalance in energy intake and energy output is the main reason for obesity because of the accumulation of fats.

Now let us see the various reasons responsible for the imbalance of energy.

In this chapter, we will discuss the various reasons that clarify the behavior of overeating and our inability to burn calories. With this knowledge, we can treat our obesity, knowingly and appropriately.

Correction of cause will lead to correction of consequences.

The nature and causes of obesity are the subjects of intensive global research, which is still ongoing. Both environmental and genetic factors are involved in the complex interaction with components such as psychological and cultural influences and physiologic mechanisms, which lead to obesity. We see that some people are obese while others remain lean. Also, it is extremely difficult to maintain the reduced weight achieved through painstaking efforts.

Various theories have been put forth to explain this fact.

Imbalances of energy inputs are generally related to factors influencing hunger, appetite or satiety.

Imbalances of energy outputs are primarily related to the thermic effect of food, physical activity and RMR.

Both energy input and energy output are influenced by heredity as well as environment.

Previously, hunger was explained as an empty space in the stomach. Then it was thought to be a drop in the blood sugar levels. Today, we know that it is our brain that feels hunger and monitors the level of our energy reserves. When these reserves get low, the brain triggers signs of hunger like salivation and a gnawing feeling in the stomach to prompts us to eat.

As our body needs energy constantly, our brain, the organ in control of our impulses and emotions, supplies the demand of energy continuously. That is why the hunger process sometimes get disrupted by strong emotions, urging us to eat when our body does not need it or conversely urging us to stop eating and starve ourselves.

Appetite is a psychological concept. It depends on the person's knowledge of food, its smell and color. Sometimes, a person tends to eat, even though he or she is not hungry. Sometimes, if the person does not like the food, he or she may not eat as the hunger dies.

Though hunger, appetite and craving are different phenomena, all of them induce a person to eat more. As a result, a person becomes obese.

We have to re-educate our appetite, by observing ourselves, between the desire of eating and actual feeding.

One theory says that distension of stomach with food gives satisfaction and one stops eating.

Another theory says that fatty food in meals satisfies the person early and for a longer time than sugary food.

Yet another theory says that lowered sugar levels lead to hunger. One more theory says that we eat to maintain body temperature. When we eat, the body temperature goes up and we are satisfied. In short, food generates heat. This is also known as thermic effect of food.

In short, very complex procedures regulate the energy intakes. After considering the complexity in energy intake, the next procedure, which is equally complex, is that of metabolism. In the metabolism process, there is the involvement of complex variables like hormonal activity, lean body mass and physical activity. Other factors such as food habits, taste, flavors, availability of food items, environment, social pressure, mental tension and psychological requirements also affect a person's food intake.

After such deep insight into the reasons why we need to eat, we can very logically say that the most important reason for obesity is **overeating**.

If the quantum of the food intake is more than what is required, then that food gets converted into fats and is deposited in the body.

If the quantum of food intake is in proportion to the energy expended, then there is not fat accumulation. Now let us see the theories related to imbalance in energy output.

As we discussed earlier, thermic effect of food contributes to approximately 10% of the total energy expenditure. The adaptive thermic effect of food, i.e. increased thermic effect due to exercise or physical activity, contributes to additional energy expenditure, which is most variable. In a sedentary individual with very less physical activity, it is 15% of the daily calorie intake. Whereas, in an active person, this value can be as much as 35%.

One of the key benefits of exercise is increased energy expenditure, above the resting metabolism rate. At the beginning, when one learns exercising, the energy expenditure is ten times higher than RMR. A trained athlete can exercise at 15 to 20 times above RMR.

This is a very encouraging fact in weight maintenance.

After an intense bout of exercise, RMR is found to be significantly higher when compared to the RMR after several days of rest.

Exercise increases demands of energy. RMR rises to meet these demands. The body then settles into a steady state of burning calories, at a rate that is greater than the resting level. The metabolism is significantly higher for 10–25 minutes and oxygen consumption remains slightly higher for two hours after the bout of exercise. Then they slowly return to a normal state.

An athlete has a higher RMR than an individual who is not physically active, i.e. sedentary. A sedentary individual can raise his/her RMR by exercising regularly without restricting calories, provided the intensity of exercise is appropriate. Low-intensity exercise cannot produce the same effect. During a bout of vigorous exercise, the muscle tissue gets slightly damaged. Its repairs as well as the glycogen required for exercising increase the metabolic cost. Also, vigorous exercise increases lean body mass, which works as an active metabolic tissue.

Exercising, Dieting and RMR

AMR is related to fat-free mass or lean mass directly. In non-exercising dieters, 24–28% of weight loss comes from fat-free mass. If a person exercises along with dieting, then only 11% of weight loss will occur due to fat-free mass. Exercise helps prevent more than 50% FFM loss.

Heredity

Most of us regularly complain that some people who constantly seem to overeat high-fat foods and sweets remain very thin, while some individuals seem destined to be obese. Many non-obese people think that only overeating and laziness lead to obesity. But nowadays, we have realized that heredity is also responsible for obesity.

Many of the hormonal and neural factors involved in normal weight regulation are determined genetically. These include the short-term and long-term regulatory signals determining satiety and feeding activity. Small defects in these signals contribute significantly to weight gain. The number and size of fat cells, regional distribution of body fat, and RMR are also determined genetically.

A study of twins having the same parents showed a strong correlation between body weight and fat distribution, while the study of adopted twins, even after feeding the same food in same quantities, showed no correlation between body weight and fat distribution. This supports the theory of genetic predisposition of obesity.

The latest study has shown that the mutant gene 'ob' is responsible for less control on the satiety center in obese people.

If both parents are obese, then 73% of their children are also obese. If one of the parents is obese, then 45% of their children are obese. Even if both parents are normal, 9% of their children are obese.

The mechanism through which genetics may affect weight gain is thermic effect of food. RMR differs from person to person. Decreased thyroid function, decreased lipoprotein lipase activity, lower body basal temperature and less amount of more metabolically-active brown fat are some of the factors responsible for a lower metabolism rate. All these factors are determined genetically. It is important to realize that genetics plays a pivotal role in the development of obesity, the rate of weight loss and weight maintenance.

But there is no need to be discouraged by your genetic legacy. If you commit yourself to a healthy lifestyle, with a scientific exercise schedule, sensible calorie control, enjoyable food habits and management of behavioral attitude, you will achieve a 100% success rate to lose weight and maintain the lost weight.

You have to remember that maintaining the lost weight is extremely difficult. When you complete your weight reduction program and achieve your targeted weight, you must be careful and not start indulging. If you indulge yourself, then you will immediately gain weight, which is more than before.

Weight Cycling

Many overweight and obese people lose and gain weight several times in their lifetime. This is called 'yoyo effect' or 'weight cycling.' With each turn of the cycle, it takes longer to lose the same amount of weight and lesser time to regain it. The weight cyclers have a lower RMR compared to normal people. Every time, during weight loss, the yo-yo dieters lose approximately 25% of their weight as fat-free mass. (which is metabolically-active tissue). This fat-free mass does not get resynthesized, when weight is regained immediately. During the course of time, it is regained. The fat-free mass supports the increased weight and movements. There is no longterm metabolic damage.

Recent study says that there is no adverse effect of weight cycling on body composition, metabolism, body fat distribution and future attempts of weight loss. However, weight cycling has a relationship with increased morbidity and mortality. Moderate weight loss grants various benefits to a significantly obese person.

Even though study shows that there is no adverse effect of weight cycling on metabolism and fat distribution, the truth is weight is lost at a slower pace, while weight is gained at a faster pace during weight cycling.

Fat cell size and fat cell numbers in obese people are different from those in non-obese people. Fat biopsy study shows that fat content within a fat cell is approximately 35% greater in obese people compared to non-obese people. The total number of fat cells in an obese person is three times greater than that in a person of normal weight.

Weight loss causes decreased fat cell diameter. The size of the reduced fat cells is somehow linked to the appetite center of the brain.

Other Reasons of Obesity

Physical exertion: Obese and overweight people are generally slow in their movements. They spend less energy in the acts of sitting, getting up and walking about. It is a recognized fact that overweight people lack necessary physical exertion. When they increase their physical activity, they increase their food intake too. But when they reduce their physical activity, they do not reduce the food intake.

In today's society, the use of gadgets like automobiles, elevators, mixers, grinders and washing machines have increased exponentially, thus reducing people's physical activity to a great extent. Nowadays, the younger generation watches a lot of TV and plays computer games for a long time, instead of engaging in some kind of physical activity.

These days, people burn 800–1000 kcal less every day than people of the previous generation. Day by day, the younger generation is becoming lesser and lesser physically active. Manual jobs and blue-collared workers are looked down upon by white collared personnel.

If a person walks 6 km in one hour, then about 400 calories are expended. Lack of simple exercise can add 1 kg every year. Rest after prolonged diseases like typhoid and hepatitis or post-operative rest leads to weight gain during the recovery period due to lack of physical activity.

Thus, it is imperative that those who wish to succeed in their efforts to lose excess weight have to increase their physical activity.

Food Habits and Digestive System

Slim children are very fussy about their food choices. They like only particular food items, while overweight children like almost all food items and keep on eating something or the other, even after meals. Obese people take big bites, eat faster and try to consume as much as possible.

Psychological and Social Factors

In today's society, people relish eating fatty dishes. This is part of an unhealthy lifestyle. It appears as though people do not eat to live but live only to eat.

This situation is created by the continuous brainwashing by advertisements that are bombarded via electronic media and hoardings and the distribution of free samples of various instant foods.

The popular perception of an overweight person is that he or she is a happy-go-lucky person, always jovial, and comes from a sound family background. In fact, such a person has no any other option but to project only this side of his or her personality. But behind the mask of a smiling face and a sense of humor lies tremendous internal conflict.

It is a very well-known fact that psychological factors play an important role in causing obesity. In fact, obesity is a psychosomatic disorder.

Food becomes a popular and easy solution for serious problems and tensions of life. People with a sense of insecurity, depression, failure and frustration generally tend to eat more and more. This activity of constant eating gives some mental peace to the person. An overweight person generally tries to develop a false sense of security by indulging in food and overeating. Many people eat when they are worried, depressed, tired, bored, irritated or excited. Many people also eat when they feel lonely or when they meet others. Some keep on eating without any reason; they just love to eat.

Food is a symbol of love, respect and warm hosting. Food is offered to guests to show one's respect and affection toward them.

It is also a well-known fact that single women, young widows and women deprived of conjugal happiness tend to be overweight. Childless couples also tend to be overweight. Transfer and transformation of happiness among human beings is done very tactfully. Sometimes, a grave psychological shock can also lead to obesity.

Those who have spent their infanthood and childhood in poverty and starvation are never able to forget or drive away their fear of unsatisfied hunger. When such people come into contact with money or wealth, they tend to eat more and more. This is the tendency of self-made personalities.

There are various types of hunger in human beings: hunger of success, hunger of relaxation, hunger of satisfaction, hunger of love and affection, hunger of social status, and hunger of name and fame. If any one of these hungers is not satiated, people tend to eat to get a physiological satisfaction of satiation.

In short, overweight people maintain their psychological balance by overeating. Gradually, they develop an addiction for sugar i.e. simple carbohydrates.

Overweight people generally present their obesity as an excuse to cover their failure and laziness. Obesity helps them avoid chores that they dislike or involve physical exertion. They make obesity a convenient excuse to avoid attending social functions, avoid getting married, and consequently avoid building a family. Once obesity takes its roots, a person begins to feel lonely. He or she may develop complexes and feel that he or she is different from others. Such a negative development adds to one's emotional problems. This, in turn, causes further obesity, creating a vicious circle. This discussion clearly brings out the truth that psychological contribution is one of the important reasons that cause obesity.

Endocrinal Gland Disorders (Hormonal Reasons)

Malfunctioning of the endocrinal glands is a cause of obesity in some cases.

In some children, Frohlich's syndrome, due to disorder of the pituitary gland, leads to obesity.

Inadequate secretion of thyroid gland brings down the metabolism of fat and causes obesity.

Cushing syndrome, due to abnormal secretion of adrenal glands, sometimes leads to obesity in middle-aged women, with accumulation of fat on the head and trunk and around the neck. In extreme cases, they become thin.

Less secretion of testicular hormones leads to obesity in men; accumulation of fat around chest, buttocks and thighs is common in this case.

In women, disorders in ovarian hormones are also linked with obesity. Weight loss is suggested as a treatment for correction of menstrual irregularities, infertility and polycystic ovarian disorder.

Due to obesity, insulin become insensitive and this leads to type II maturity onset diabetes. Weight loss can reverse the disease in an early stage. Some experts say endocrinal disorders lead to obesity, while others say obesity leads to endocrinal disorders.

Metabolic Disorder in Obesity

Do metabolic disorders lead to obesity or does obesity lead to metabolic disorders? This is a great challenge for researchers.

When some people consume excess food, a lot of heat is generated in their bodies. This utilizes the food in the body. Consequently, their weight remains constant.

Whereas, some people do not have the capacity to generate heat to utilize the food consumed by them. They tend to gain weight. Food is the only source of fats. The fats consumed get deposited in fat stores and made available whenever required.

When excess proteins and carbohydrates than what is required are consumed, they get converted into fats. This process occurs generally in the liver. However, organs like intestines, lungs, heart, spleen, and diaphragm can also transform carbohydrates and proteins into fat.

The body metabolism of obese people does not deal effectively with carbohydrates. Carbohydrates are catabolized only to a certain extent (that is up to the pyruvic acid) and then they are converted into fat. Thus, production of fat through carbohydrates is an additional feature. Whereas elimination of fat is at a very low level. In short, for an obese person, carbohydrate is also a source of fats.

Some scientists do not agree with the above-mentioned theory. According to them, consumption of excess food than required is the reason for extra fat deposition.

Frequency of meals is also an important aspect of metabolism. A person who eats one heavy meal has a high level of glucose. This leads to the production of a high level of insulin. This is responsible for fat formation. The habit of taking a heavy meal at late evening or night leads to more fat formation, as we have seen that the rate of metabolism is slow in the later part of the day.

Small and frequent food intake does not lead to too much fat formation.

When simple carbohydrates are consumed in large quantity, they lead to high levels of glucose and insulin, which drop down the metabolism rate. The process of utilization of food slows down and this leads to production of fats. When more proteins and fats are consumed, BMR goes up and food utilization rate increases. This is the reason why we must cut down on carbohydrates, especially simple carbohydrates, and increase the protein intake in adequate quantities, to prevent the BMR from dropping.

There are differences of opinion about the issue of BMR in obese and normal people.

Percentage of Fats in Men and Women

The size and strength of muscles in women are different when compared to men.

Men have stronger, heavier and more musculature than women because of the male hormone testosterone.

Women perform the function of reproduction. Female hormones support this function by contributing more fats for the childbearing age, from menarche (from the onset of monthly periods), during pregnancy, till menopause. During the various stages of childbearing period, which is approximately 35–38 years, many women keep adding fats.

In men, the fat percentage is 15–19% of the total body weight. In women, the fat percentage is 21–25% of the total body weight.

Some Uncommon Reasons for Obesity

Quitting smoking leads to weight gain.

Side effects of some drugs like anti-depressant (like Amitryptiline): These drugs stop the shedding of accumulated fats and increase the weight. This increases carbohydrate craving and thirst.

Sleep-inducing drugs like chlorpromazine cause weight gain.

You must have understood that you overeat for various reasons, even if you are physically inactive. The reasons behind your behavior have various origins.

In the next section, we will see the psychological status of obese people and learn to overcome every hurdle before starting treatment. With a clear mindset, we shall proceed further.

Section II

Psychology and Health Screening

- Health behavioral psychology
- Screening and health assessment
- Benefits of weight loss

Chapter 5

Psychology of Obesity and Weight Management

Introduction

In the first section, we read about what obesity is, body composition, the effects of obesity on our health and the causes of obesity.

By now you may have decided to undergo a correct scientific treatment for weight reduction and weight maintenance. Intellectually, you have agreed to do this weight reduction program by changing your lifestyle and accepting a new and healthy lifestyle.

To accept such changes forever, one needs special mental and psychological preparation. Do you know that obesity is a psychosomatic disorder? Your psychology plays an important role in becoming obese and in getting treated for obesity. It is extremely important to learn the psychology of weight maintenance and obesity. The study of the psychology of weight maintenance helps in prevention, treatment and identification and evaluation of the factors that optimize overall health.

Your behavior, such as overeating and remaining inactive, is due to various psychological reasons.

Let us gain some knowledge about the reasons of behavior related to weight management and modifications, if required.

This will help you accept the changes forever, so that maintaining the reduced weight becomes easier.

All of us are very much aware of the benefits derived from weight loss by leading a healthy lifestyle. But many of us do not adhere to a healthy lifestyle. Why it is so? Let us examine what motivates us and what is required, so that we can make permanent changes in our behavior.

Trans-Theoretical Model

If you have been physically inactive for many years, i.e. if you like to read, watch TV, play video games, surf the net, watch movies or chat with friends in your leisure time, then it is very difficult to change these habits and start participating in exercises, sports, trekking and walking. It is challenging to transform from a chronic (long lasting) unhealthy behavior to a stable and healthy behavior. Accepting this challenge and making it happen is a lengthy process involving several stages. Psychologists have developed the transtheoretical model for behavioral change. The underlying processes to change unhealthy behavior and adopt healthy behavior are described in the stages of change.

This model is very useful to change health-related behavior like physical inactivity, weight control, nutrition, smoking, stress and alcohol abuse.

During the various stages of this model, if we apply specific behavior change techniques, the rate of success for change increases. Understanding each stage of this model will help you determine where you are in relation to your personal healthy lifestyle behavior. It also will help you identify techniques to make successful changes.

Read the following stages and see where you stand/fit in.

Pre-Contemplation

In this stage, one does not want to change the behavior. One does not accept any problem and one denies the change. The individual is not aware or is less aware of the problem. Other people, including family, friends, healthcare practitioners and coworkers, identify the problem of behavior easily. The individual does not know, does not care to know, and does not want to know his behavioral problem and may avoid any information and material that addresses the issue.

Such an individual avoids free screenings, workshops and lectures that could help identify and change the problem, even if he or she receives financial incentive for attending them. The individual frequently and actively resists any change and seems resigned to accepting unhealthy behavior as 'one's fate.'

It is very difficult to make these individuals accept that there is a very grave problem in their attitude toward behavioral change. They think change is not possible at all. Educating them about the behavioral problem is critical.

Friends and family of such individuals, who are concerned about them, must remember that knowledge is power. With correct knowledge of the consequences of obesity, others can make individuals realize that they are ultimately responsible for the consequences of not changing their behavior like physical inactivity and perpetually eating the wrong kind of food. The help of other family members, friends and seniors is very important. In case the individual in question is a child, then a teacher or any other person who influences the child's decision-making can be involved. Sometimes, the person initiates a change only under pressure from others just to make others happy.

Contemplation

During this stage, people acknowledge that they have problems and begin to seriously think about overcoming them. They start thinking about the pros and cons. Yet, they are not quite ready to change.

They may remain in this stage for years but they keep planning to take some action within the next six months or so.

It is the responsibility of the well-wisher to educate the person about obesity, its treatment and its consequences. Well-wishers must support the person without getting tired or angry and create positive pressure.

Preparation

During this stage, people are seriously considering and planning to change their behavior in the next month. They take initial steps for change (such as exercising on weekends) and may even try them for a short period. They define the general goal of behavior change and write specific objectives to accomplish this goal.

The role of the parents, family, friend or well-wishers is extremely important. They have to give company to the person during exercise. They have to take his or her commitment for the next session, discuss positive consequences and health benefits, and make available healthy, nutritious, low-calorie and tasty food. They also have to give company while the person is eating. Their comments like 'I feel very light and fresh after eating this food' will make the person realize that he or she has the same feeling.

Action

This stage requires the total commitment of time and energy on the part of the individual. Here, people actually start practicing the things required to change the behavioral problem actively. They do the things required to adopt a new healthy behavior. The person starts the exercise designed for him or her and the diet planned by the dietician. Many times, the person may regress to the previous stage. Optimum guidelines help give positive results. You need to help the person get the correct prescription.

Relapse is generally common. The action stage should be maintained for six consecutive months. Only then one can move on to the maintenance stage. During the action stage, others have to appreciate the efforts of the person and acknowledge him or her even if there is very little progress. Others should admire the consistency of the person. After three months, the person can be made to realize the improvement in fitness level. He or she may be rewarded to encourage him or her. The most important thing is to bring to notice the health benefits the person has achieved.

Maintenance

During this phase, the person adheres to the behavioral change for up to five years. During this phase, there is a continuous adherence to changed behavior like low-cal diet, regular exercise and engagement in a game, which will improve the physical activity of the person. During this stage, the person reinforces the gains made through the various stages and strives to prevent lapses and relapses. The individual enjoys a slimmer figure than before and starts wearing properly fitted clothing. There is an improvement in health status, confidence level boosts, and self-esteem increases.

Termination/Adoption

After a period of five years, the termination or adoption stage happens, without the fear of relapse. In case negative behavior is exhibited, the stage is called 'termination.' If a person adopts positive change for more than five years, then this period is called the 'adoption stage.' Now there is no obstacle in the healthy lifestyle and we can say that the person has achieved his or her goal.

Principles of Behavior

If you keep repeating the same pattern of behavior, the behavior becomes a habit. Unconsciously and automatically, you keep practicing the same behavior. To break the habit, you have to learn how you formed it.

Antecedents, i.e. stimuli that lead a particular behavior, are the triggering factors. If you habitually eat popcorn at movies or eat chocolate and *chikki/toffee* after a meal, you will always remember popcorn when you think of movies and you will get restless without chocolate or *chikki/toffee* after a meal.

Consequences may be positive or negative. Positive consequences increase the behavioral recurrence. Negative consequences have the opposite effect. If you eat Chinese food and get a stomach ache, the next time you may not have Chinese. On the contrary, if you enjoy a wonderful dinner with your friend at a newly opened restaurant, you will plan to visit the place again.

Many times, there is a **behavioral chain**. You get tired or frustrated and buy a pastry. Then you feel guilty. After a few hours, you tend to eat two bowls of ice cream. Not buying pastry in the first place would be an easier step to take than battling the urge to binge when you feel frustrated and tired.

Shaping behavior is the reinforcement of successive approximations until the desired goal is reached. A child may refuse to have fruits during break time in school. But he or she starts showing readiness if you teach him that vitamins and minerals will give him power like Superman, while eating bakery products may lead to diseases.

Listening to the same story every day helps shape behavior, leading to the final goal of accepting nutritious food.

Observational Learning

Social environment, which provides models for behavior, can affect your behavior.

For example, Salman Khan's gym workout can be effective for your adult son who has recently joined the gym.

Current thoughts, feelings and cognitions can function either as antecedents or consequences for overt behavior, thus influencing your action in a manner similar to environmental events. Feeling lonely may trigger eating episodes that lead to guilt.

With proper knowledge of these principles, we can decide behavioral strategies for weight control and lifestyle management.

Behavioral Strategies

- Stimulus control method

- Substitution of incompatible behavior

- Behavioral contracts

- Rewards

- Cognitive methods

Stimulus Control Method

If you are an overeater, you decide the timings and specific place at home for eating. For example, you may decide this: *I will eat only at the dining table and only at specific times like 8 a.m., 1 p.m., 4 p.m., and 7 p.m.*

You will find it very difficult initially. Triggers to eat will eventually pop up. If you are habituated to eating while watching TV, sitting on your sofa, you will initially get irritated by this new resolution. But over a period of time, the triggers lose their power and the target behavior extinguishes itself.

Substitution of Incompatible Behavior

You have to substitute your misbehavior with an alternative good behavior. Instead of watching TV, you can take a walk, play a musical instrument, sing a song, read a book or do any other activity that is not related to eating.

Contracts

It helps a lot if you write an agreement specifying your targeted behavior, the frequency and timeline, with the consequences as conditions, and sign it with your caretaker, loved one or consultant.

For example: I will be very regular for my workout this week between 6.30 a.m. and 7.30 a.m. I am not going to eat anything beyond the advice of my dietician. So, I will lose at least 400 grams of weight this week.

Rewards

Rewards have positive consequences. You reward yourself when you achieve any change in your misbehavior. Even simple praise from others encourages a person to adhere to the changed behavior. Try to reward a person who is trying very hard to change his or her behavior with a token gift. Rewards may not be expensive but they should have a symbolic value. Acknowledgment from others is more influential than the reward itself.

Cognitive Method

Any event or misbehavior leads to a thought and a thought then leads to a reaction. Such thoughts could be guilt, anxiety or worry. People link their self-worth with their achievements. So, do not set any unrealistic, maladaptive or extreme goals. Sometimes, if you eat something that you are not supposed to eat, do not blame yourself. Instead try to get back to the prescribed low-cal diet immediately.

We have now gained brief knowledge about behavioral strategies. Let us learn the basic methods to adopt the changes in behavior.

Basic Methods to Adopt the Changes

- **Assessment** is essential to develop appropriate and effective intervention plans.

You can assess yourself with the help of a consultant. You must provide all information about your weight history.

Forget your previous failures during the treatment. Make a fresh beginning. Neither criticize previous treatment nor compare the results or pattern, even if it is the same or different. You have to be determined to do the program successfully and maintain the lost weight permanently, come what may.

You may want to join the program because of pressure from family to get married or get a better job. You may be in a dilemma or think that you would do whatever you find convenient. Then, before starting the program, it is better you have a clear discussion with your consultant. You have to do the program for yourself. Learn about the health risks associated with obesity. Be open to accepting your misbehavior, which needs to be corrected immediately.

Have discussions with successful people who have lost weight and are maintaining the same. Insist on group meetings with successful people. Start the program only if you are ready to change and give your 100%. Do not join any program under peer/social pressure. Get a clear-cut idea of what you are supposed to do. Try to learn the basics of nutrition in a simple way. Learn the basics of exercise science in simple words and only then start the treatment.

You have to anticipate and set aside time for attaining the required results. Be clear of the amount of efforts you have to invest in the program. Unrealistic goals will make you unhappy and give you a feeling of failure, which may demotivate you.

Learning

You have to learn how to implement your diet and exercise plans.

The first step is to set the goal. (Refer to the part on goal setting at the end of this chapter.)

Get a clear-cut idea about the ideal weight you should have and the realistic weight you can achieve.

Do not do overload yourself. For instance, do not plan to exercise for more than 60–70 minutes a day.

The plan must be **scientific.** This means the diet should be balanced and you should avoid starvation and fad diets. Do not skip any meal in a day. The exercise must be scientific, systematic and safe, neither above nor below your fitness level.

The plan must be **systematic.** You must have a thorough idea about how to perform exercises and what the constituents of your meal should be.

The plan must be **progressive.** Exercises should be learned step by step.

The plan must be **concrete.**

The plan must be **cohesive.**

Food shopping, habits, emotions, exercise, food choices, portion control, timing of meals and snacking must be planned. Strategies like meal scheduling, deciding the place for food, nutrition education and stress management are really helpful. Triggers for eating must be identified, so that control techniques can be planned. The program must not be painful or difficult; only modifications in the existing food pattern will be helpful and adaptable to your daily routine.

Always add variety to the meal and exercises to avoid boredom. Self-monitoring is important. Maintain a diary of the exercises and diet and plot a graph of the progress. This is helpful to learn your body's response to particular foods, particular timings and particular exercises.

Other family members can support you by giving company while eating and during exercise. Nutritious eating is useful for everyone. Even if others are not giving you company or they eat whatever they want, you have to stick to your program by keeping in mind that you are doing the right things and others are following the wrong things. Eating fruit and not cake is always better for anyone. Cake is junk and our stomach is not a dustbin to be dumped with junk often. You have to train your taste buds for the right food and develop a taste for the correct nutritious diet. You can add spices, try out various recipes and make the food tasty. Even though other family members may sometimes be troublesome or discourage you, you have to be strong enough to adhere to the program you have selected. You derive strength through self-help and support groups in your social circle or from your consultants. Or you can take the lead to form such a group with the help of your consultant. You can engage in fun social activities with yourself and incorporate simple and funny games that will improve your physical activity. You can have competitions for low-cal recipes and engage in discussions on the problems you face during weight loss. Anonymous overeater groups will help you as well as others who are sailing in the same boat.

Overeaters anonymous are a group of people who share the same problem. They will help combat isolation, boost your confidence in your changes, and enhance your motivation. When everybody in the group shares their experiences, their progress stories and their difficulties, it will act as a source of useful information regarding effective change techniques.

It is vital and essential that this group performs all its activities in the presence of a trained weight loss consultant, so that if anybody has lost weight through any unscientific method and shares their experiences with others, the consultant can intervene. This way others can be prevented from getting tempted by useless or dangerous information, which is not based on scientific evidence. The weight loss consultant will guide people to stay away from such harmful methods of weight loss.

As a participant in the group, you have the capacity and conviction to discuss scientific techniques with confidence. This will help you adhere to your treatment strongly and others will also get benefited. You will be admired by the consultant and the other participants too. This will help you follow your weight less program more religiously and rigidly.

If you are a person concerned with somebody's weight loss, then you have to form a support group to encourage the person to stay on track. Compliment the person on his or her efforts and remark positively on the success made. Do not be a source of sabotage, discouragement or frustration for anybody who is trying to lose weight. You must offer your help and provide valuable suggestions.

Always review your progress to evaluate your behavior so that you are appraised of your behavioral change. Such a review will help you analyze the quantum of your efforts. If you find yourself putting in less efforts in the implementation of weight loss plan, you will be determined to put in extra strenuous efforts.

For instance, if you observe your previous month's diary, you may notice a pattern: you had lost 3 kg while exercising for one hour a day and you had stuck to your diet plan meticulously. Whereas this month, in the last 15 days, you were not regular in your exercise and you had to attend two parties. Therefore, you did not lose even one kg of weight. This review will reinforce your faith in the weight loss plan and you will start following the plan more rigidly.

Remember: Act in a new way of feeling rather than feel yourself in a new way of acting. Self-monitoring is an effective, standard assignment. It provides continuous feedback and opportunities for self-correction.

Try new strategies, write down the objectives of new exercises and diet plan, find a source of social support, brainstorm with your consultant when your body is not responding, think of alteration of plans and social events, and make a list of personal rewards after reaching short-term goals.

Keep on evaluating and monitoring the change in your measurements or clothing size. Assess your feelings moving from 'good' to 'better.' Study your fitness measures and health benefits like change in blood pressure, sugar level and changes in eating pattern. This will provoke your behavioral change. This will help you review your progress and learn critical lessons. It will help you watch out for signs of relapse and other warning signs. It will also give you an idea of the things that are really helping in the weight loss and those that are not.

When you monitor your progress, you will know the techniques you can continue while maintaining your weight. You can repeat the diet plan that gave you best results. For example, having legumes instead of sprouts might have given you a better rate. In case you tend to relapse, that is you come to the baseline, keep discussing with your consultant. Get a redirection. Look at relapse as an opportunity to finetune your technique. Do not get disappointed or frustrated when there is a relapse. Do not feel you are a failure, do not give up. Learning is a process that does not occur at a constant rate, in a constant direction. Slips are normal and they provide good learning opportunities. Keep in mind the example of a baby learning to walk. It needs a lot of help and it falls down a lot. But it does not get discouraged, it keeps on trying to walk until it succeeds. No one tells the baby to forget walking.

During a weight loss program, it is common to do it halfheartedly and follow whatever is convenient. You may also feel like giving up the program for a social reason like a party or a gathering.

Ask yourself the following questions to evaluate adherence during a month:

How many situations you had to go away from your plans?

What are the barriers in the plan?

Are you overloaded?

Are you feeling as if you are failing?

Are you frustrated?

Are you feeling less confident?

Do you feel you have to do lot for achieving a small gain?

There are two important guidelines when addressing adherence. Always attend to those things you are doing well, not just the problem areas. Secondly, make sure you are having realistic expectations. Work optimum to achieve a successful experience.

For a successful lifestyle management program, you have to understand your abilities. You have to have awareness of personal limitations. As discussed many times earlier, your misbehavior alone is not responsible for your obesity; other health problems or medical conditions like hormonal imbalance, psychological disorders, and low performance in exercise due to coronary or pulmonary problems could affect the direction of your program. In such a case, you have to consult your physician or a medical expert to design your program at an optimal level.

In the chapter on health assessment and screening, we will discuss the conditions in which we need to consult a psychotherapist.

All the principles for weight loss and weight management can be summarized in the following manner. A detailed behavioral pattern can be reformed thus, for our day-to-day activities.

1. Stimulus control

A. Shopping

- Shop for food after having meal.

- Shop as per the list.

- Avoid ready-to-eat snacks.

- Do not carry more cash than required for shopping. This will stop you from buying tempting readymade foods.

Always think this: *I am going to eat nutritious, low-cal food. Readymade food is junk. I am developing healthy habits with which the quality of my life will improve.*

B. Plan

- Plan to limit food intake.

- Substitute exercise for snacking.

- Eat meals and snacks at a scheduled time.

- Don't accept food offered by others.

Don't say 'yes' when you want to say 'no.' Denying food humbly will not insult anybody. This will give the idea that you do not eat outside your schedule. This is good for your health. Eating junk is not good for health, even though some people may not have a problem of being overweight.

C. Activities

- Store food out of sight.

- Eat food at the same place.

- Remove food from inappropriate areas in the house.

- Keep serving dishes off the table.

- Use smaller dishes and utensils.

- Avoid serving food to others.

- Leave the table immediately after eating.

- Don't save leftovers.

- Don't participate in the preparation of food, to avoid the temptation to eat while cooking.

- Don't eat out of the plan.

- Make the 'allowed' food always available and the 'not allowed' food unavailable.

Do not give room for any temptation. Food is for you, you are not for food. Eat how much is essential and whatever is necessary. Stick to this, no matter what.

D. Holidays and parties

- Avoid alcoholic beverages, soft and hard drinks.

- Plan eating before the party.

- Eat low-cal snacks before the party.

- Practice a polite way of declining food.

- Do not eat just because others are eating.

- Wear good clothes and jewelry, have a good time, share good jokes, keep telling yourself about your successful efforts to lose weight, discuss positive changes, participate in dancing and singing, and be cheerful throughout the party.

- On holidays and festivals, plan group walks, water aerobics, group games and good competitions. Read books and write your experiences. Go to the beauty salon or get massage treatments. Clean the house, write letters to your loved ones and enjoy the day in a fabulous way. Find out ways that will keep you active, happy and help you remain on your diet plan.

2. Eating behavior

- When you have a mouthful of food, wait till your mouth is empty before you take another bite.

- Chew 32 times till the food gets converted into liquid paste.

- Don't keep the food plate empty.

- Eat slowly.

- Pause in the middle.

- Do not watch TV or read while eating as it lowers the metabolism.

- Enjoy the food selected as per your plan. Do not think that you are eating fodder. Think that you are eating vitamins, minerals and fibers, which will reward you by improving your health.

- Do not get irritated if anyone forces you to eat junk prepared by them. Humbly explain to them how it is not useful to health and how it is harmful to you and anybody and everybody who eats that.

3. Rewards

- Solicit help from friends and family.

- This support should be in the form of praise or token gifts.

- Use self-monitoring records to prove your progress as a basis for rewards.

- Plan specific rewards for specific achievements.

- Plan some rewards for change in behavior even though you are yet to reach the complete level of achievement. Getting a pat on your back, either from others or yourself, will motivate you further.

4. Self-monitoring

- Keep a diet diary that includes the time, place, type of food, quantity of food and your mental attitude.

- Note down who was present with you when you were eating and how you felt.

- Maintain an exercise card with the details of the type of exercises, number recorded, repetitions, and timing on the tread mill.

- Note down the weight before exercise and after exercise, the measurements when you started exercises, and the measurements every three months.

- Make a record of the last plateau.

- Record the food and exercise pattern during the plateau.

  ➢ If you are a woman, make a note of the premenstrual weight, weight during periods, weight with contraceptive pills, and weight after menstrual period.

Premenstrual Syndrome

An average of 5 out of 10 women may suffer from some physical or emotional distress during the premenstrual phase (before you get your monthly periods).

The following symptoms may be observed:

- *Bloated abdomen and fingers*

- *Swollen and tender breasts*

- *Weight gain from 500 g to 3 kg*

- *Headache, often on one side*

- *Aching back, legs, shoulders, knees and ankles*

- *Craving for sweets, high-carb food*

- *Pimples, boils, spontaneous bruises, clumsiness, dizziness and fainting*

- *Exacerbation of asthma, epilepsy (convulsions).*

Emotional symptoms include:

- *Tension and anxiety*
  - *Depression*
  - *Tearfulness*
  - *Forgetfulness*
  - *Lack of concentration*
  - *Irritability*
  - *Inability to make decisions*
  - *Violent mood swings*
  - *Lethargy*
- *Loss in confidence*
  - *Disinterest in sex, work and social life*

The above symptoms have to be managed with an action plan.

- *Try to plan your life so that you do not put yourself under premenstrual strain.*

- *Reduce water retention by reducing sodium intake.*

You can restrict sodium by avoiding table salt, processed food like chips, pickles and, papads. Substitute them with fresh salads, vegetables and fruits.

- *Do not worry about temporary weight gain. It is the weight of retained water, which you will lose during your menstruation.*

- *Keep food craving in check. If you gain weight because of fulfilling the craving, then you will not lose it after menstruation.*

- *Lift your mood by attending concerts, movies or play.*

- *Take up yoga, relaxation techniques or meditation to relieve tension.*

- *Take extra care if you are prone to exacerbation of any health condition.*

- *Do some aerobic activity followed by stretches.*

- *Develop awareness of symptoms and try to exert self-control.*

- *Do not use any vitamins or drugs without consulting your physician.*

- *Do not treat this period as an excuse to put on weight.*

- *Keep a record of your behavior.*

  ➤ *Be active, divert your attention and seek medical help if required.*

Menstruation is not a condition you are facing alone. Every woman undergoes this cycle. But have you seen the women athletes? How do they maintain their calm and do rigid and strenuous physical activity? You must train yourself to accept menstruation as a natural phenomenon.

5. Nutrition education

- Use a diet diary to identify the problem areas.

- Make small changes that you can continue.

- Learn the nutritional value of foods like *poha*, upma, porridge and other snacks that may seem light but are high in calories. Understand about the empty calories that junk and bakery products contain. Learn about simple carbohydrates, sugars, jaggery, honey, alcohol, *sarbat* and soft drinks. They can raise your weight remarkably. Honey is believed to help in weight reduction. Well, read the chapter on nutrition thoroughly. Also refer the calorie reckoner in Appendix.

- Minimize fat intake.

* Consume more fresh vegetables, fruits, fiber-rich food and complex carbohydrates.

6. Physical activity

- Increase your routine activity.

- Use the staircase instead of elevators.

- Avoid vehicles for short distances.

- Start walking your dog.

- Try to get down from the bus one stop earlier and walk the rest of the distance.

- Engage in a game or go around the ground.

  ➢ Walk instead of watching TV, reading or playing videogames.

- Learn dancing, swimming or aqua aerobics.

- Take an interest in hobbies that will make you mobile.

7. Exercise

Do the optimum amount of exercises. Avoid under-exercising or over-exercising. Keep a record. Notice your progress and modify your workout, if need be. Progressively increase your exercises as your fitness improves.

8. Cognitive restructuring

- Avoid setting unrealistic goals.

- Think of progress, not shortcomings.

- Avoid words like 'always' and 'never.'

- Counter negative thoughts with rational restatements.

- Set weight goals.

- Follow the recommendations for maximizing exercise adherence.

General principle: Be sensitive to psychological and physical barriers. Keeping a separate hall for obese people can make them comfortable. Availability of clothes in your size can give you the assurance that there are people of your size in the world. There is no hard and fast rule that you should wear track suits or leotards while exercising. You can use any comfortable clothes that will allow you to do exercises without difficulty.

Start with simple exercises, they will improve your efficacy. In the initial days, try to be mobile. Then learn to maintain your pace. Slowly elevate your program to a higher intensity.

Be consistent, enjoy the routine. Don't look at the time constantly to see if you will complete the entire prescribed exercise routine. It is important not to waste your time by watching yourself in the mirror or chatting with your neighbor.

Compliance is important.

Do not try to compensate overeating by increasing your exercise.

Take into consideration your body's limitations.

Form a group and encourage each other while doing the exercise.

Specific Interventions

Get clear information about the importance of exercise.

Be physically active throughout the day.

Give your 100% for each count.

Start self-monitoring, feedback and goal setting techniques.

Identify other benefits like physical change, increased mobility and lower resting heart rate.

If you are under any emotional distress, choose exercises that soothe instead of choosing overeating as a remedy, which in itself is a high-risk factor.

Increasing Program Adherence

How you approach your program of weight loss decides your adherence to it. Make it clear to yourself that the behavioral changes are for the lifetime. You cannot store the results you achieved with your efforts. You have to maintain them with your changed life style. **It should not be a program of weight loss like losing 10 kg in 25 days**. It is a reshaping of your habits for life.

It is not a 'diet' and 'exercise program,' it is commitment to a **healthy lifestyle** forever. Whether you have tried such a program many times before or you are trying it for the first time, you have to accept the lifestyle change permanently.

Most people opt for an excessive approach by skipping meals or doing exercise for 3–4 hours. Then the program becomes burdensome to continue for them. Three meals a day and one-hour exercise with an active lifestyle is the recommended change. Otherwise, you will not be able continue the burdensome changes; then weight cycling takes place. You have to develop a healthier, personalized pattern with the help of an expert, which fits sensibly into your daily routine. This will increase your adherence to it. A busy woman who works full-time will find it difficult to work out for two hours or a physically inactive man will find it difficult to start a hardcore program.

Assess your fitness, take the advice and supervision of experts. Allot only one hour for exercise, keeping in mind your routine. You should feel energetic throughout the day, not tired or sick, when you start your exercise regime.

Frequently monitor the effectiveness of the plan in terms of results, the rate of progress and the effectiveness in fitness level.

How to Deal with Setbacks?

If you are not experiencing the desired level of success, it may be due to intentional or non-intentional-non-compliance of the program or due to a biological link that you have inherited genetically. You have to find out the reason. Discuss repeatedly with your consultant, give him or her a clear idea of your intake and output. Do not get frustrated. Get more and more knowledge about your body and your treatment.

Lapses are an inevitable part of the weight loss program. Take them as tools of understanding your body. Understand the reason for the lapses. Learn how to deal with such a situation the next time it happens. Lapses can be overcome by self-monitoring, whereas relapses happen after many lapses. You either return to the program with vigor or get frustrated and drop out. Both lapses and relapses teach you about your strengths and weaknesses. You will learn from these experiences. When these happen, you must seek professional help. Then you will realize that it takes time to achieve the goal. You will understand the importance of a scientific program.

The risk factors for lapses and relapses

- Negative emotional stage

- Motivational level

- Response to treatment

- Coping skills

- Social support

By understanding your risk factors, you can cope with setbacks. Lapses are due to situational factors; relapses are due to personal negative emotional status, such as depression.

It is important to review your initial reaction to the program. It indicates how you will proceed further. Many times, even if you do well in the beginning and you are 'perfect' to start with, you may relapse later. If you have a mindset that you can have lapses and relapses, you will perform better by accepting the program as a lifestyle change.

You have to know about eating disorders like anorexia, bulimia and binge eating, which are discussed in the next chapter.

Chronic dieters keep going on and off the diet plan. They are under risk of developing an eating disorder. **Exercise abuse** is also a category in which people who keep thinking about exercises all the time; it becomes compulsive for them to exercise. Such people feel anxious if they miss even one session. They think about weight gain constantly. Even though they are injured, they keep doing exercise. If they overeat, they exercise. They keep thinking about the calories they have burned. In such a case, psychiatric help is necessary.

Transforming the body to the ideal weight is an unrealistic goal. Efforts to reach it can be taken to such an extreme level that it may lead to the point of emotional distress or psychological problem. During your weight loss program, you have to take the help of a consultant, you have to discuss your problems with your consultant. You have to accept the program as a lifestyle change forever. Breaks in between should be considered normal and you should try to stick to the change in spite of them. Set realistic goals and try to achieve them. You have to make the program successful, for which you may even have to take the help of a psychiatrist, if required.

Study of behavior psychology gives you a clear-cut idea of your mindset and helps you achieve progress, by giving ideas of your shortcomings and strengths. You are unique. So, you need a plan that is uniquely designed for you, specifically. Compete with yourself, compare with yourself, and try to be better tomorrow than yesterday, with regard to your behavior, plan and progress.

Motivation and Locus of Control

Why do some people succeed and others do not? Motivation often explains this. Although motivation comes from within, external factors trigger inner desire.

People who believe they can control any event in their lives are said to have an internal locus of control. People who feel that chance and environment are responsible for controlling events in their life are said to have an external locus of control. The people with external locus of control have a difficult time accepting the treatment for weight loss. They feel powerless and vulnerable.

If you are from this category, if you feel environment or external factors are responsible for your overweight, you have to develop an internal locus of control. Then you can change your lifestyle and adhere to exercise, a changed diet plan and a healthy lifestyle. Understanding that most events of life are not determined genetically or environmentally help people pursue goals and gain control over their lives.

The **three factors** that can help you enter the preparation stage are: competence, confidence and motivation.

1. **Competence:** You may not have skills in all activities. This leads to less competence. You can select the activity in which you are skilled. Don't be afraid to try new activities. If you cannot do aerobics, you can participate in simple circuit training. You can try several new low-cal new recipes, which are good in taste.

2. **Confidence:** When there are skills with no belief and conviction, maybe because of fear or feelings of inadequacy, this interferes with the ability to perform the task.

   Try to visualize yourself doing the task and getting it done. Repeat it several times and then give it an actual try. You will surprise yourself by doing the task very easily.

   If you feel that the task is too hard to do, divide it into smaller realistic objectives to make it simpler. If you need to lose 25 kg, you must target 5 kg in the first two months. Perhaps you can do the task in 40 days; this will boost your confidence. You will learn some skills in physical activities. Losing the next 5 kg will perhaps be simpler for you. If, on a given day, you cannot accomplish the task, don't give up. One day, you will complete it.

3. **Motivation:** Sometimes, in spite of competence and confidence, you may not be willing to do anything. Perhaps lack of knowledge is the reason for this unwillingness. Knowledge often determines goals and goals determine motivation. Are you unaware of the consequences of overweight? Do you lack the knowledge that stroke, heart attack and cancer can be irreparable or lead to fatal consequences of obesity? Get more and more knowledge about the consequences; this will help you stay motivated.

Old habits die hard. You need continuous efforts to change your wrong food patterns. Sooner the implementation of a good pattern, greater are the health benefits. Not only will you lose the weight but you will also enjoy the quality of life.

Make a list of the good consequences of a weight loss program and the bad consequences of being overweight.

Do an analysis of diet. Where you are failing? Are you eating *khari* and biscuits with your morning tea? Do you like *vada samosa* for breakfast? Do you consume *laddoos* after a meal? Find out the timings, the quantity and the type of high-calorie food consumed during your daily diet. Simultaneously, find out the timing when you really waste an hour watching TV or remaining in bed. This will help you set the goal.

A goal motivates change in behavior. The stronger the goal or desire, the more motivated you will be. You have to prepare the action plan accordingly.

Find a supportive circle of friends who really help you by admiring your achievements. If you lose 5 kg, the friends must tell you that you are looking great and younger by five years. They are your real friends. The persons who say you are looking sick or you may regain fast should be avoided.

The best solution is for you to monitor your progress yourself. The weighing scale is your real friend; it shows you all the minute results of your efforts. Continuous monitoring of your weight and measurements by keeping a daily record of your intake and exercise will encourage you to maintain the plan systematically. It also helps you know what diet helped you lose weight efficiently. How is your body responding to a particular change in exercise? What should be your pattern to achieve maximum outcome? Does eating more salads and vegetables help you? How efficient is this?

Monitoring encourages you to eat right and work out right. You get proper appreciation from your weighing scale. If the weighing scale is showing less, then you should not worry about what your so-called friends say.

You have to have a positive approach from the beginning and believe in yourself. Try to imagine how healthier you will be in future.

Even though, in between, you may not get good results in spite of your sincere efforts, you must try hard. You must control your calories and be efficient in exercise. Even if the weighing scale does not show the desired figure, do not get disappointed. Many physiological factors, like water retention, contribute to such results. You deserve good results for your good efforts. Do not worry; perhaps your weighing scale will show an expected figure within a period of week.

Learn chapter 3 – energy expenditure TEF. Weight plateau.

To once again get a clear-cut idea about energy metabolism.

If you do not feel like rewarding yourself, try to meditate. Practice sincere efforts and keep thinking that if not today, tomorrow your desired weight would be shown by the scale. Keep telling yourself this: *I am giving my 100%, my body will also show 100% results. I am improving my fitness, I am looking better. I am on my way to success. I will reach the goal.* Such self-reassurance helps a lot; it gives you the strength to continue. When you overcome the plateau, reward yourself in a better way.

Goal Setting for Change

To initiate change, goals are essential. Goals motivate behavioral change and provide a plan of action. Goals are most effective when they are:

1. **Well planned**: I have to lose 3 kg in the first month. For that, I will follow a diet plan as per the guidelines of my dietician. I will regularly exercise as per the guidelines of my instructor.

2. **Personalized** goals are easier to achieve. Your mother may want you to lose weight quickly, but you decide your own pace.

3. **Written:** An unwritten goal is a wish; a written goal is a contract. Show the written goal to your consultant, trainer, dietician and friends. Do not fight alone. Take the signature of someone on your written goal.

4. **Realistic:** Goals should be within reach. Ten kg in 25 days and a 3-hour exercise regimen every day are nonrealistic, unscientific goals. At times, even the attainment of realistic goals becomes difficult. You decide to go for a walk and suddenly it starts raining. You have to change the plan and do some indoor activity.

5. **Measurable**: 'I will lose weight' is not an adequate goal. You have to decide how much to lose in what span of time. This is important. *I want my waist measurement to reduce to 34 inches in 4 months. I want to lose 1 inch per month.* These are measurable goals.

6. **Time specific:** The goal must have a specific date for completion. Make this date realistic; but let it not be too distant in the future.

7. **Monitored:** Diet diary, exercise log, fitness measurements, body circumference and body composition assessment will help you.

8. **Evaluated:** Periodic re-evaluation is vital for success. If you reach the goal before time, it means you have probably set an easy goal to achieve. Therefore, you have to set a higher goal. If you cannot reach the goal you set, in spite of your efforts, you have to reassess the goal. Once you achieve the goal, set a new goal to improve or maintain your efforts.

If you are motivated, then you have to find out the right time to start the program. Are you starting the program immediately because of your poor physical health? Are you feeling depressed? Are you being pressurized by your spouse, parents, friends or coworkers? Are you hopeful of improving your social life, getting a good life partner, or getting a promotion in your job? If such is the case, you feel that immediate results will be beneficial to you. Then indeed this is the right time to start the program. But if you are under pressure or if there is a lot of stress at work or the stress of studies, then you have to wait till you get enough time to focus on the weight-loss program.

Once you decide to start the program, then plan for sensible and reasonable weight loss. Do not begin the program with a burst of enthusiasm that may fade. Once the rigor of the program sets in, the commitment is for lifetime. Otherwise, you will have to face problems like weight cycling, feelings of failure and decreased self-esteem.

Once you decide to begin the program, the first step is to set the goals as discussed earlier. While setting the goals, you have to take into consideration how genetics play a role in this weight and weight-loss program.

After setting the goals, keep in mind that some goals can be achieved easily, while others may take time.

We have to consider the short-term and long-term psychological goals that have been often associated with losing weight.

Short-Term Psychological Goals

- Weekly goals for problem areas: For example: *This week, I am not going to have bhel chaat when I am with my friends. (Or) I will avoid sweets after lunch and dinner.*

  ➤ Keeping a record of emotions before and after eating: For example: *I can control my feeling. Even though I like vada, pakoda, cutlet and patties, they are not good for my health. Let me eat only one. I will not even touch it. Salads are really boring. I am feeling like a saint. I feel like crying. I am feeling proud as I can control myself. Raw food fruits are improving my digestion. My skin is getting better, I am feeling great. I will lose like yesterday. I feel I have lost one inch around my tummy. At least for one month, I will give my 100%.*

  ➤ Practice assertive requests, setting limits and sharing feelings. For example: *Actually, till yesterday, I gave you company for alcohol but from today I will not drink, at least for one week. I will not eat at this party, but I want to chat with everybody. I will have fruit instead of karanj/deep-fried sweets, I am sure I will be successful.*

- Engage in activities that have been avoided due to weight or negative body image. You can dance or participate in group discussions. You can try the clothes you like.

Long-Term Goals

Improved self-esteem

Improved problem-solving abilities

An understanding of the connection between problem eating, unwanted eating and emotions

Ability to communicate with anybody about your weight-control plan

When you achieve these goals, you will become psychologically strong, you will improve your confidence and you will follow the treatment more happily.

You have to remember that everyone has some problem or the other. Even though others feel that obesity is due to your laziness and overeating, now you are aware that there are other physiological and psychological factors responsible for this problem. This is a disease and you have to get scientific treatment for it. Some people have to fight with arthritis, some have to face asthma, likewise you have to face obesity.

You have to plan a logistically sound treatment program. Before starting the program, you have to do health screening and assessments to make the program safe for you.

Chapter 6

Screening and Health Assessment

Introduction

We have learned that there are many factors that influence a person becoming obese. Before starting the treatment, it is necessary to identify the underlying contributors for your obesity. Many times, we may need the physician's assistance or psychiatric consultation before starting the treatment. Sometimes, if a person has some health condition like anorexia, weight reduction is contraindicated. To rule out any contraindication, screening is important.

With assessment of health, you can design the framework of the treatment plan. This makes your program safer. If required, you can get the physician's advice to get surety about safety, which helps you adhere to the program.

Before starting the actual treatment, let us learn about screening for your suitability for the treatment, assessment of relevant medical and psychological factors, along with the fitness parameters—to know whether you require the assistance of a healthcare professional. In addition, information that is collected during the assessment phase provides an important foundation for establishing a safe and effective treatment plan for you.

Obesity is a serious threat to health and wellbeing. Medical risks associated with obesity, like diabetes, hypercholesterolemia, gall bladder diseases, hypertension, cancer and cardiovascular diseases, are life-threatening. The economic, medical and psychological costs that our society has to bear are staggering. Many individuals are now attempting to control their weight. However, weightloss treatment, if not taken up scientifically, can lead to serious health problems. In some cases, there are contraindications to lose the weight, i.e. in some peculiar cases, the doctors would advise the obese patient not to lose weight. Thorough screening and assessment of an individual is extremely necessary before starting the treatment.

Nowadays, there are various options of treatments available for weight loss. But choosing the wrong option would prove very harmful to your health. This may be the result of your lack of knowledge about the most scientific and non-harmful option for weight loss.

For the safety of your health during weight loss, you must think seriously about the safest ways to follow.

Follow these Awareness Norms Strictly

- *Warning – Rapid weight loss may cause serious health problems (more than 1 kg per week).*

- *Only permanent lifestyle changes, such as making helpful food choices and increasing physical activity, promote long-term weight loss.*

- *Before starting any weight-loss program, take the advice of your family physician.*

- *Treatment like exercise and diet plan should be taken from a qualified professional.*

- *When you have decided to take the right treatment, you have the right to get thorough information about the treatment like price, products used, medication, supplements, tests, program duration, risks associated with the program, rate of weight loss, and future plans to maintain the lost weight.*

You are supposed to get a low-fat diet from a qualified professional and suitable exercises from a trained person. You have to ensure that the person giving advice and treatment to you is well qualified. You can lose weight safely. You have to learn to maintain it as well.

If your age is above forty years, you are a sedentary person or you have a particular history relating to health, then you have to take medical advice before proceeding to the next step. If, as per medical advice, certain dos and don'ts have to be followed, you have to follow them under the supervision of a trained person.

If your weight is more than 30% above the normal weight or if you are facing some medical problems related to your weight, you have to take the help of a physician for supervision of your program.

If you are 100% overweight, then your treatment has to be intensive, with a very specific diet, medication, psychotherapy and, if necessary, surgery. In such a case, it is extremely dangerous for you to start your treatment with any non-professional center without any medical advice.

Do not take the decision influenced by any advertisement. Do not think about looking good alone, think about getting healthy and fit. Health must be prima facie; weight loss must be the byproduct of your changed lifestyle. With your changed life style, you are going to get a fit body.

Do not compare yourself with any model, hero or friend. Compare yourself with your old, obese, unfit, diseased self and feel happy that you are better than yesterday and you will be even better tomorrow. Compete with your own self. Achieve the new milestones of getting more mobile, getting better strength, stamina, endurance and flexibility, improving fat percentage, improving self-image and self-esteem. Feel proud about your achievements. Reward yourself. You are marching successfully toward your goal of fitness and health by following a very tough and hard path. Now you are ready to start your program. You have to get your physical health assessed by your physician.

If you do not have any significant current or past medical problems, then it is sufficient to record the following vital aspects:

Height and weight

Body mass index

Waist to hip ratio

Blood pressure and resting heart rate

Current medication

Chronic illnesses

Medical history

Family health history

Health-related habits – cigarette, alcohol, drugs

With the help of the above information, your counselor can assess your fitness and identify and record risk factors that you may or may not be aware of having.

Set a realistic goal after a brief discussion with your consultant. It is very important to discuss your previous efforts at losing weight, your dream weight, your ideas about ideal weight, your readiness or difficulties to follow the treatment part, any possible modification in your diet or exercise plan and if you find it difficult, your personal likes and dislikes and so on.

Do you have the habit of starvation or fasting? Do you sometimes feel like eating uncontrollably? When you are disturbed, do you satisfy yourself by eating? Do you feel very low about your physique? Do you keep thinking that you are looking extremely ugly? Do you compare yourself with your competitors? Do you get disturbed if anybody suggests that you lose weight? Do you feel that you miss out on many opportunities, good friends, good company or success at work due to your obesity? Are you seeking a program that will give you fast results without exercise or a diet plan? Are you just ready to pay without working hard? Do you have ideas about losing weight by just popping tablets, drinking juice or having medicine after eating whatever you want? Do you feel that, without anybody's help, you cannot do any workout? Do you feel lonely when you start any weight-loss program? Do you continuously keep thinking about your body image? Do you feel shy, ashamed and less confident? If you are willing to discuss all your problems briefly with your consultant, then he or she can help you overcome them? He or she may help you directly or guide you to take the help of a psychotherapist.

There is nothing wrong in taking the help of a psychotherapist. Obesity is a psychosomatic disorder. Many times, managing the somatic treatment part helps manage the psycho treatment part.

And many times, psycho treatment helps manage lifestyle change. Many psychotropic medications such as anti-depressants, anti-anxiety pills or mood stabilizers may facilitate or hamper weight loss significantly.

Certain psychological conditions like anorexia nervousa, bulimia nervousa and binge eating disorder, are contraindications to start the weight-loss program. A person with depression needs to get psycho treatment prior to weight-loss treatment. During depression, an individual experiences pervasive feelings of sadness, hopelessness, helplessness and worthlessness. There is sleep disturbance too; either one oversleeps or does not sleep at all. Eating difficulties like overeating or lack of eating, excessive guilt, fearfulness, cry spells and difficulty in concentrating are also common. Combination of exercise and medication helps overcome depression. If you experience any of the above problems, then you have to discuss them with your consultant, prior to starting the treatment. It will help you overcome your problems as well as your obesity. For this, it is important to have knowledge about eating disorders.

Anorexia Nervosa and Bulimia Nervosa

Anorexia nervosa and bulimia nervosa are seen typically in members of middle-class families. Unresolved conflict is the general cause for these diseases. Middle-class families value slimness a lot. At the same time, food is used for recreation, survival and health. The developmental problems of affected individuals make them extremely vulnerable to these mixed messages. Gorging and vomiting, with or without starvation, is seen. This is called bulimia. About 50% of anorexic patients develop bulimia. Characteristically, anorexic patients refuse food. About 25–35% of weight loss is seen in them. They exercise vigorously, may abuse laxatives and diuretics, and vomit without a break. This disorder progresses to starvation. It is very important to recognize the symptoms of anorexia at an early stage. The important symptoms are:

Fat store depletion

Muscle wasting

Amenorrhea (absence of monthly period)

Desquamation (soreness in mouth)

Dry skin

Hirsutism (presence of hair on face)

Thin, dry and brittle hair

Alopecia (loss of hair)

Degradation of finger nails

Postural hypotension (giddiness while changing posture)

Dehydration

Edema (swelling)

Bradycardia (decrease in pulse rate)

Hypothermia (feeling cold)

Constipation

Sleep disturbances

Bodypnea (body pain)

Anorectics have an abnormal fear of being fat, which is exhibited in distortions of body image and other perceptions, probably reflecting a combination of altered physical state, distorted perception and denial of perception leading to self-gratification. Such patients experience arrested development. They do not develop a normal sense of self or a complex and advanced pattern of thinking.

Bulimics try to restrict food intake, which is less than a normal person's diet. They feel that they have eaten a lot and try to purge by vomiting or with laxatives. Physical complications like damage to teeth, irritation of the throat, inflammation of the esophagus (swelling of food pipe), cracked and damaged lips, and broken blood vessels in the mouth are due to repeated vomiting and vomiting efforts. Overdose of laxatives leads to rectal bleeding, dehydration, electrolyte imbalance (particularly low values of calcium), kidney damage, and muscular diseases (these can be corrected with treatment). Bulimics have a normal weight but they are afraid of gaining weight. They do not feel self-worthy even when they gain a little weight and they suffer from psychological problems like inability to face frustrations and guilt, over-binging and vomiting, even when their lives may seem ideal to those around them.

Anorectics turn away from food, bulimics turn to food. Anorectics may present as perfectionists and conscientious and confirming adolescents, while bulimic anorexics may demonstrate rebelliousness, emotional instability and impulsiveness. Bulimic patients compulsively eat to avoid painful problems and then get fearful about weight gain. They feel ashamed of their 'out-of-control' behavior and attempt to remove the food from their bodies before it can be absorbed.

Binge eating disorder (BED): A person with this disorder decides to diet in the pre-condition phase. One gets an uncontrolled desire to eat in the triggering phase. Yet one maintains a low-cal diet in the maintenance phase, then loses control, and eats at least ten times more than the normal diet in the ending phase. Finally, one feels distressed in the post-binge phase. Binging is common in dieters.

The binge eater is often obese unlike anorexic or bulimics. The binge eater does binge eating at least twice a week.

Generally, 30% of individuals seeking weight-loss treatment suffer from BED. You have to ask yourself the following questions, which will help you know whether you suffer from BED or not.

- Were there times during the day when you could not stop eating even when you wanted to?

- Do you ever find yourself eating a large amount of food in a short period of time?

- Do you feel extremely guilty or depressed afterwards?

- Do you ever feel more determined to diet or eat healthier after the binge eating episode?

In case you experience any of the above symptoms, you should opt for psychotherapy along with the weight-loss treatment. In the presence of anorexia, weight loss is not recommended at all. Bulimia and BED require psychotherapy before, during and after treatment of weight loss.

Assessing Exercise Readiness

If you do not have any health complaint or wrong habit, then you can start your exercise and diet program without the physician's consultation. The intensity of exercise should be moderate i.e. well within your current exercise capacity, can be continued for 60 minutes, and is non-competitive.

If you are a woman who is over 50 years or a man over 40 years, even if you do not have any health complaint, you need to get the physician's approval to do vigorous exercise. Vigorous exercise can be explained as the exercise in which intensity causes mild to moderate breathlessness or results in fatigue after 20 minutes of exercising.

If you have any history or complaints but do not have any symptoms, then you can start a moderate-intensity program without the physician's approval. But you cannot do any vigorous exercise before a medical exam. If you have symptoms that are suggestive of any disorder, then you should not start even a moderate exercise program before your medical and exercise tests. Even during the exercise test, physician's supervision is required.

Assessing Fitness

Under the guidance of professionals, with all the safety measures in place, you can start a moderate exercise regimen. After a period of three months, it is advisable to undergo a physical fitness test that will help you assess your fitness level after three months of moderate exercise in relation to age and sex. Theoretically, it is advised to assess the fitness level at the beginning of the program but if you are sedentary, you may get the wrong message that exercise tests are strenuous, you lack physical fitness, you need to take crucial care and your limits are too much. Therefore, the assessment of the fitness has to be done at the end of the three-month period of moderate exercise. This is very helpful in the following areas.

- In development of exercise prescription

- To identify areas of health and injury risk and the need for possible referral to a healthcare professional

- To establish realistic attainable goals and provide motivation

- To get educated about your physical fitness

- To evaluate the success of the fitness program through follow-up assessments.

Though you may feel frightened or embarrassed to undergo the assessment, keep in mind that minimum evaluation will provide safety, confidence and readiness for exercise.

Readiness to Change

Now it is time to assess whether it is the right time to make a serious attempt at losing weight. Readiness to change is a complex phenomenon that will help find your motivation to lose weight, your commitment to restructuring your life, and your current life circumstances. If your readiness is high, you will be successful.

Even though you feel that you are not fully committed to losing weight, many times, your motivation increases when you enjoy some success and witness the benefits of a changed lifestyle. Many times, your readiness to change your lifestyle is merely superficial enthusiasm or an inborn wish for your lifestyle to be different. Strong commitment to persistence is needed to make the change possible.

In case of pregnant and lactating ladies who want to lose weight, the advice of a gynecologist is very much required. In case of people with anorexia or an underweight history, a psychologist consult is needed along with the physician's advice. In case of obese children, advice of a mental health specialist may be required. Bulimic eating disorder and other psychological disorders require the advice of mental health specialists. Significant cardiovascular renal or medical problems require a clinical weight-loss program.

When you start your weight-loss program and you feel any symptom related to your health occurring in between, you have to seek medical advice regularly from your physician. Keep informing your physician, trainer, weight-loss consultant and dietician about any medical findings.

If you are doing a weight-loss program with an institute that has access to healthcare professionals, do seek their advice, as they are always updated with the latest knowledge about weight loss, exercise and nutrition and will be able to relate them with your conditions. This will boost your confidence and morale. Many times, you have to take the lead and insist to your physician and your weight-loss consultant on having a periodic discussion about your weight, your program, your progress and your future plan. Your sincere effort will make the program safe. Get yourself screened for your suitability for the program, get your fitness parameters and medical and psychological factors assessed, and seek the advice of allied health professionals if there are any indications. After all, you deserve an effective weight-management program.

Chapter 7

Benefits of Weight Reduction

Introduction

The encouraging news for the population that is trying to lose extra weight is that even 10% of weight reduction can lower the risks associated with health. It lowers blood pressure, improves glucose levels, reduces risks of heart attack and strokes, decreases sleep apnea, reduces signs and symptoms of arthritis, and improves the general status of health.

This encouraging news will motivate you to maintain whatever weight you have lost and lose further weight till you reach your dream weight. Now, commit yourself to a healthy lifestyle to become disease-free and healthy.

Lose Weight and Gain Health

Weight loss has been found to improve a number of medical problems associated with obesity. To avail yourself of such benefits, it is not necessary to wait till you get to the ideal body weight. Even during the first phase of weight loss, you can accrue many benefits.

- Control of diabetes: Calorie restriction and exercise improve the ability to use insulin and normalize blood glucose levels. Obese diabetic patients, after losing 10–20% of their weight, can often reduce and sometimes even discontinue the use of diabetic medication.

- Improvement in hypertension: Weight loss has been found to improve blood pressure. Long-term weight loss of even 5% is sufficient to significantly reduce blood pressure. It allows the patient to discontinue the use of antihypertensive drugs. Dietary changes help reduce blood pressure, with the help of healthy eating habits, such as a low-sodium and reduced-fat diet. Exercises cause capillarization. This leads to more number of capillaries with a good distribution of blood volume. Due to exercise, blood volume gets distributed to the extremities on a large scale. Reduction of the total surface area reduces the work load. This leads to better management of blood pressure.

- Weight reductions from 5–10% often results in large reductions in serum cholesterol and triglycerides. Recent reporting is that weight reduction of 11% leads to 23% reduction in serum cholesterol and 16% reduction in triglyceride. With exercise, good cholesterol HDL increases.

- Menstruation problems like dysmenorrhea i.e. painful monthly cycle, amenorrhea i.e. absence of monthly cycle and other irregularities in menstruation get corrected after weight loss. Many cases of infertility get good results after weight loss. In poly cystic ovarian diseases, weight loss is a suggested treatment.

- Even though all cases of infertility cannot be treated, married life becomes enjoyable in general. Impotency due to obesity in men and frigidity due to obesity in women disappear and people start enjoying a satisfying marital relationship.

- Weight reduction reduces the undue burden on weight bearing joints viz. hips, knees and ankles in particular and all joints in general. There is a considerable relief in pain as stiffness of the joints vanishes and movements are restored. Chances of osteoarthritis are done away with. With a 10-kg weight loss, the knee joints get a longer lease of life by 10 more years. Patients get relief from backache. Exercise strengthens the muscles and connective tissues, leading to improved supporting system of the joints. Bones also get stronger and denser due to exercise. This helps in prevention of osteoporosis (brittleness of bones), which leads to frequent fractures in later age.

- Weight reduction helps in the management of hernia.

- Weight loss also helps in prevention of varicose veins.

- Weight loss causes reduction in perspiration, which is a social gain as well.

- The skin develops resistance to infection.

- Psychological and social gains: You develop a better physique, an important aspect of your personality. This leads you to overcome any inferiority complex. Self-respect, self-esteem and self-confidence improve and social life becomes enjoyable. Generally, obese and overweight people are targets of fun and ridicule. They are denied a life partner and a good position in their career. Such problems are solved through weight-loss programs. Exercise improves posture, gait, strength and overall fitness, while a good diet improves the luster of skin and the glow in the eyes.

- Good fitness leads to a reversal in the aging process.

Do not get discouraged due to misconceptions about weight loss.

- You will not feel weak. On the contrary, your fitness improves because of exercise. You will not get tired.

- You will not look sick or old. On the contrary, with a balanced diet, you get good and proper nutrition. Your energy levels go up.

- You feel young and you look young. You experience youth and feel/appear younger than before, due to increased lean body mass, increased bone density, increased stamina, increased flexibility, improved cholesterol levels and increased hemoglobin.

- Your skin will not look loose and flabby as it gets enough nutrition. Due to exercise, the blood circulation toward the skin increases.

- Your digestive system will not get weakened. On the contrary, taking enough proteins and consuming all vegetables will improve digestion. Fibers remove problems like constipation.

Do not get discouraged by the wrong arguments put forth by friends, family members or colleagues. Get the advice of your physician and you will realize that scientific weight loss will give you good health, beauty and looks.

Section III

Lifestyle Management through Healthy Lifestyle

Introduction

Congratulations! You have educated yourself about obesity, with the most current and complete knowledge. Now, with this perfect mindset, you can learn about the treatment for obesity.

As we know, there are several reasons that lead to obesity. But the permanent solution for weight reduction and weight maintenance is just one. It is lifestyle management through a healthy lifestyle. A healthy lifestyle is a multifaceted approach to weight loss and weight maintenance. It involves the following:

- *Scientific exercise regimen: 'Scientific' means 'safe and effective'*

- *Sound and balanced nutrition*

- *Good rest and relaxation*

- *Positive mental attitude*

- *Commitment to a healthy lifestyle: It will not only help you lose weight but will also ensure you maintain the weight you have reduced.*

In addition to weight loss, you will get a quality life. Health is the prima facie evidence of the lifestyle management program; weight loss, beauty and quality of life are the byproducts of a healthy lifestyle. What else do you expect? So, get ready to fight obesity to gain health.

(The permanent solution for weight reduction and weight management)

- Exercise

- Basics of nutrition

- Diet principles for weight loss

- Rest and relaxation

- Positive mental attitude

- Weight maintenance

- Approaches to be avoided

- Prevention of obesity

- Low-calorie recipes

- Frequently asked questions

Chapter 8

Exercise

Introduction

Exercise is an extremely important aspect of a healthy lifestyle. During the weight-reduction program, exercise is extremely essential. It prevents loss of valuable fatfree mass during weight reduction. Only unwanted fats get lost, which is a requirement of weight reduction. For effective weight reduction, we have to learn the scientific exercise regimen, which comprises resistance training, aerobic training and flexibility training. Let us learn the science of exercise and avail ourselves of all the benefits mentioned in this chapter.

Exercise is elixir! Even though you are not obese, you have to exercise. Without exercise, you cannot have a quality life. One hour of exercise a day must be a part and parcel of your life.

When you are determined to change your lifestyle and commit yourself to a healthy life style, it is very important to understand about scientific exercise regime, which is the first important aspect of your new lifestyle. Exercise is the closest thing to the miracle pill that everyone is seeking. It brings in weight loss, appetite control, improved mood and self-esteem, energy revitalization and a longer life by decreasing the risks of heart disease, diabetes, stroke, osteoporosis and chronic disabilities.

Research has established that participating in a lifelong exercise program contributes greatly to good health. If you perform fitness tests after regular exercise, you will find that you are well conditioned as you had dreamed. To reap significant benefits, the basic principles of exercise have to be followed essentially. For optimum results, the program must be individualized. Personal needs and fitness levels vary from person to person. The basic principles of exercise in general and for weight control with maintenance in particular are presented in this program. With this exercise regimen, you will promote and maintain physical fitness and wellness along with weight loss.

Dieting never has been fun and never will be. People who are overweight and are serious about losing weight will have to make exercise a regular part of their lives, along with proper food management and perhaps a sensible cut in caloric intake. As discussed in the previous chapters, some precautions are necessary. Depending on the extent of the weight problem, a medical examination, possibly a stress test or an ECG (this is described in detail in chapter 6 on screening and health assessment), should be done.

Significantly overweight persons have to choose activities in which they will not have to support their own body weight but will still be effective in burning calories. Injuries to joints and muscles are to be avoided by not participating in weight-bearing exercises such as walking, jogging and aerobics. Initially, the activities that should be incorporated are cycling, water trading, resistance training with very moderate weights and more repetitions. They will assist you in losing weight without pain and fear of injuries.

Exercises allow the fat to be burned more efficiently. Both carbohydrates and fats are sources of energy. With prolonged exercises, glucose levels begin to drop and more fats are used as energy substrates. Fat-burning enzymes increase due to exercise.

Initially, muscle glycogen store is utilized for energy production, which is required for exercises. Thereafter, as the concentration of the enzymes increases, the ability to burn fat also increases.

As we have already discussed in chapter 3, we are aware that, compared to high-intensity exercise, exercise with moderate intensity burns more fats because of prolonged lactic threshold. The more moderate is the intensity, the higher is the percentage of fat utilization as a source of energy. The intensity should not be too low as well. The total calorie expenditure within one hour must be optimum, so that the total daily calorie expenditure exceeds the calorie intake. The intensity should be increased as your fitness goes up. As the intensity increases, your metabolic rate remains at a higher level and it triggers greater fat loss. Your goal is to reach a high intensity by conquering small goals with moderate intensity. When you gradually build up your fitness level, you will be able to participate in a high-intensity program. But do not attempt too much too quickly.

At any cost, safety is the priority. You have to avoid injuries and discouragements. After proper conditioning of 8 to 12 weeks or even longer, you can think of high-intensity training, provided you are moderately overweight. If you are extremely obese, then aim to achieve body conditioning through proper resistance training. Gain strength in the muscles and achieve agility, balance, and improvement in efficacy. Only then can you switch over to a moderate-to-high intensity exercise regimen. This switch has to be done with continuous trials.

Keep in mind that you have to follow low-intensity exercises at the beginning, to avail yourself of all the health benefits and to increase your capacity to participate in moderate-intensity programs—so that you can burn more calories than before and gain more fitness. Finally, you can reach a high-intensity training regimen to enjoy maximum benefits and improved calorie burning. If your body does not allow you to go for higher intensity, you can increase the duration of the exercise period, after the conditioning phase of 8 to 12 weeks.

Scientific Exercise for Weight Loss and Weight Maintenance

You have learned that a scientific exercise regimen is the first important aspect of a healthy lifestyle, which you have committed to.

Scientific exercise is a combination of:

- resistance training with gym exercises

- aerobic exercises or cardiovascular training

- stretches or yoga exercises for flexibility(Paragraph is over)

Gym Exercises for Resistance Training

After your health screening and assessment of body weight, height, body mass index, body measurements from ankle to neck (with proper techniques described in anthropometry), you are ready to march on the path of your goal of weight loss and maintenance. Your trainer will escort you till you reach the goals safely.

The trainer takes into consideration the present status of your physical fitness, your limitations and your plus points. Accordingly, he or she will design a program especially for you. Everybody has to follow a tailormade program designed based on one's fitness level and other aspects. The exercise schedule should move from light to heavy, simple to advanced, and easy to hard to make your body adapt to changes and progress accordingly.

Resistance training is based on two basic principles: progressive overload principles and specificity of training.

The fitness components, namely strength and endurance of your muscles, follow the principle of 'use or lose.' If you use your muscles in the proper way, you can strengthen them with a specific technique. If you do not use them properly, they will lose their strength. If muscles cells are overloaded beyond their normal use with additional resistance, then the cells will improve their capacity to exert force in terms of load. If you will overload the muscle cells, with a number of repetitions performed with moderate resistance, they will improve their capacity to do more repetitions. This is endurance. If demands decrease due to sedentary work or rest for any specific condition like long illness or post-accident recovery, the cell strength decreases and so does the endurance.

The overload principle states that to improve muscle fitness components like strength and endurance over time, you have to increase resistance to a significant magnitude to produce development in the muscles. (Weight or resistance should be viewed in terms of dumbbells, barbells, machines or body weight). Muscles have to be taxed beyond their accustomed loads to increase the physical capacity.

Specificity of training means a specific type of training is given for a specific purpose of fitness. For weight loss, we are going to concentrate on improving the endurance and strength components of physical fitness.

Muscular system is the machinery of our body. Stronger the machinery, greater is the fuel consumption. Stronger the machinery, more efficient is the work done. This means, if we improve the strength of our muscles, they will be able to burn more calories. Then we can perform our daily tasks very efficiently and effectively. With resistance training, we can improve the strength of our muscles and the endurance of our muscle cells, through a specific mode, resistance, sets and frequency of training.

For weight-loss program, everyday endurance training without much rest in between the sets is recommended to preserve muscle mass and prevent muscle loss during weight loss. Fat loss is the target. The workout must be able to provide the benefits of aerobics and resistance training. During the first month, your weight is more and you cannot perform aerobics. This is to avoid stress on weight bearing joints. Endurance training with cardiac equipment like treadmill, cross trainer and cycle and endurance strength training with a set of 20 repetitions help in fat loss and prevent muscle loss.

The duration of the workout should not be more than 65 minutes and less than 55 minutes for weight loss. Over-training in terms of resistance, frequency and duration has to be strictly avoided. Under-training is also not recommended.

Beginners, sedentary individuals and elderly persons should get rehearsal practice with low resistance and more repetitions. The principle of 'light-to-heavy, simple-to-hard, less-to-more' is very important.

Many times, individuals seeking weight loss are unable to do even a simple activity. In order to make them mobile, we recommend very simple exercises like moving their extremities at the possible range without any resistance. Slow marching, slow walking and machine exercise with very light resistance and more repetitions are recommended. Within a period of 4–6 weeks, they gain confidence and slowly they start the normal workout properly.

Following are the guidelines for strength training during weight loss:

- You have to select exercises for all major muscle groups.

- You should not do the exercises alone. Always do the workout with a trained instructor.

- Warm up properly with some light-to-moderate aerobic activity and a few stretches, prior to resistance training.

- Exercise large muscle groups (chest, back, legs, hips) before you exercise the small muscle groups (arms, abdominals, ankle, neck).

- Exercise opposite muscles groups for balanced workout. When you work the front thigh (quadriceps), you have to work the hamstrings i.e. back thigh as well.

- Perform the exercise in a controlled manner. Avoid fast and jerky movements and do not throw the entire body into the lifting motion. Do not involve the lower back or neck by maintaining a natural curve of spine by avoiding arching.

- Do each exercise through the entire range of motion.

- Do not hold your breath while lifting resistance. Inhale, i.e. breathe in, while lowering down the weight and exhale, i.e. breathe out, when you lift the weight up.

- Do not hold the breath while lifting and straining. This increases the pressure in the chest, abdominal cavity and blood vessels.

- If there is any unusual discomfort or pain, stop the exercise immediately and inform your instructor. If he or she allows you to continue, you may proceed.

- Stretches of every muscle group is important.

Signs of Over-Training/Over-Exercising

- Aches and pains persisting throughout the day

- Tired feeling and inability to sleep well

- Loss of appetite and loss of body weight

- Lower immunity to cold and sore throat

- Lack of motivation during workout

Requirements of Good Workout

- Each set must be challenging.

- The whole workout should make a person feel that he/she has given maximum effort.

- Over-exercise must be avoided at all the costs.

- Under-exercise is better than over-exercise.

- But consistent under-exercise will not accomplish desired goals/results.

- Under-exercisers usually drop out of the program due to boredom or lack of visible results.

Strength training in a weight-loss program is designed in such a way that your endurance and strength increase. Simultaneously, you will accrue the benefits of aerobic exercises of very moderate intensity. It will not exert any undue pressure on your body or your mind. It improves your confidence and fitness level. The most important thing is that it will improve your adherence to the exercise, which is an important aspect of a changed lifestyle.

Benefits of Resistance Training

Gym Exercise

- **Strength:** *It improves the strength of muscles, bones and connective tissues. Strength is the important component of fitness. It can be described as the capacity to exert maximum force to do maximum work and is measured as one maximum repetition. When you overload your muscles with resistance, in terms of repetition and weight load, the muscle cells adapt to this new challenge by increasing its size i.e. hypertrophy in males and strength in both males and females. Your muscle cells become stronger. Within a period of three months of proper training, you can realize that you can lift more weight.*

  The muscles having their origins and insertions in bones through tendons and bones are connected to each other with ligaments. The impact of strength training is further forwarded to the bones and connective tissues. With regular workout, they get stronger.

- **Endurance:** *Endurance is the capacity of the muscle group to perform the same work again and again, with moderate resistance. With regular resistance training in the gym, you can improve your endurance. The 15 repetitions that were very difficult on the first day of workout become easier after a month of regular workout. When this component of fitness enhances, your capacity to cope up with daily task improves. You do not get tired at the end of the day and you feel energetic throughout the day.*

- **Flexibility:** *In gym exercise, we contract our muscles to lift the resistance. When we do the exercise of a particular muscle (prime mover or agonist), we contract it concentrically and the opposite muscle (antagonist muscle) contracts eccentrically. This helps improve flexibility. In addition to this, after resistance training, we always perform stretches, which again help improve flexibility.*

  Flexibility is the capacity of the muscles to get stretched to achieve full range of motion around the joint. Every joint has its maximum range of motion. When we improve our flexibility, we can use the maximum range of motion. This helps avoid injuries.

- *Gym exercises, i.e. resistance training, help in maintaining the recommended body weight and body composition. Your muscles and bones become stronger, your lean body mass improves and your calorie-burning capacity enhances. The stronger muscles burn more calories, even at rest. The thermic effect of exercise burns more energy. Your total body fat percentage starts reducing. These exercises help achieve weight loss. They change your body composition toward the ideal fat percent.*

- *Gym exercises improve the resting metabolism rate. This is a result of increased and stronger lean body mass.*

- *They enhance the posture and physical appearance. Resistance training includes all major muscle groups.*

- *Regular exercise improves strength, alignment and flexibility of all body parts. Muscle tone improves, adding beauty to your physical appearance.*

- *Your confidence level boosts. Improvement in physical strength leads to improvement in your psychological strength as well. You start looking better. Straight stretched shoulders and back and less fat around the tummy, hips and thighs improve your self-image, self-esteem and overall personality. Improvement in your personality and your physical fitness improves your motivation and adherence toward the changed lifestyle for the maintenance of the lost weight and to enjoy life.*

Weight loss can be accelerated by combining aerobic exercises with a strength training program. Each additional kg of muscle tissue can raise the BMR by 70 calories per day. If you add 3 kg of lean body mass, with the help of strength straining, you will raise the BMR by 210 calories per day, which equals to 10 kg of fat loss per year. When strength training is combined with aerobics training, the calorie expenditure increases.

If your weight is extremely high, then you have to start with non-weight-bearing aerobic activity like cycling, water trading or water aerobics.

If you are moderately obese, then you have to consider a whole-body workout at your own pace in the beginning and then low-impact, low-intensity aerobics. After a period of 8 to 12 weeks, you can participate in a moderate-intensity workout.

You have to take care you don't overload your muscles for development.

Aerobic Exercises

The word 'aerobic' means 'in the presence of oxygen or with oxygen.' When we start exercising, the demand for oxygen increases but as the body does not respond so quickly, there is deficit of oxygen in beginning. As the heart rate (HR) starts going up and the heart starts pumping more blood, the increased demand for oxygen is slowly met. Enough oxygen is now supplied at the muscle level. Energy production at the muscle level is done in the presence of oxygen. This is called aerobic production of ATP as energy. During aerobic exercise, all body parts and muscles are supplied with enough oxygen. This increases the heart rate.

During aerobic exercises, there is a stimulus to the cardio-respiratory system, by making the heart pump faster for a certain period of time. Cardio-respiratory development occurs when the heart is working between 40% and 85% of the heart rate reserve (HRR). For unfit people, beginners or obese people, the training intensity should be 40% of HRR. Slowly, you can reach up to 85% within a period of 12–24 months. This will help increase the maximal oxygen uptake. You have to follow the dictum of 'slow and steady' in the beginning.

You can calculate the intensity of exercise by simple methods. You have to learn to monitor your pulse either on a radial artery (on your wrist, under your thumb) or on a carotid artery (on your neck at either side, near the vocal cord under the jaw).

To determine the intensity of exercise or cardio-respiratory training zone, follow these three steps.

- Estimate your maximal heart rate (MHR) by the formula 220 minus age (220 – your age).

- Sit quietly for 15 to 20 minutes. After some time, check your resting heart rate (RHR) after some time. Check it for 1 minute.

- Determine the heart rate reserve (HAR) by subtracting resting RHR from MHR (MHR – RHR).

- Calculate training intensity (Tl) i.e. 40%, 50%, 60% and 85%. Multiply it by HAR and then add RHR to it.

- For example:

  If your age is 20,
  MHR = 220 - 20 = 200 beats per min (bpm).
  If RHR = 68 bpm
  HRR = 200 - 68 = 132 bpm
  40% Tl = (132 x.40) + 68 = 121 bpm
  60% Tl = (135 x.60) + 68 = 147 bpm
  85% Tl = (132 x.85) + 68 = 180 bpm
  Low-intensity cardio-respiratory training zone is 121–147 bpm.
  Moderate-intensity cardio-respiratory training zone is 137–157 bpm.
  High-intensity cardio-respiratory training zone is 157–180 bpm.

If you are physically inactive and you have to start an aerobic workout for weight loss, you have to maintain the heart rate between 40% and 60% intensity for at least 8 to 12 weeks. Slowly, you can increase the intensity. At a low intensity, your metabolic profile will improve. After achieving 60% to 85% intensity, you can achieve a 'good' or an 'excellent' cardio-respiratory fitness rating. Maintaining this will help you maintain a high fitness level.

Do not go above 85%, as, with this intensity, you will neither avail yourself of the benefits nor will you be safe. Weight-loss clients should not exceed 65–75% of TI.

Mode of Exercise

Aerobic exercise has to involve the major muscle groups of the body with rhythmic and continuous movements. More the muscles involved in the exercise, more is the effectiveness of activity providing cardio-respiratory development. Exercises like walking, cycling, swimming, climbing stairs, stationary running and cycling are aerobic exercises. These activities should be enjoyable. Your physical limitations must be taken into consideration while selecting the appropriate mode of aerobic exercise. In any case, you have to avoid high-impact activities. Weight-loss clients should do strength training with low resistance and more repetitions for 12–16 weeks, prior to a low-intensity aerobic activity with low impact. This reduces the incidence of injury significantly.

Duration: 30 to 40 minutes of moderate-intensity exercise followed by 10 to 15 minutes warm-up can provide substantial benefits. 10 minutes of exercise at 70% MHR thrice with a four-hour interval also provides fitness benefits. If you do not have one hour to spare, you can work out three times a day as per this advice. A cool-down session of 5 minutes is a must after any exercise.

Frequency of exercise: Three to five sessions per week are recommended.

For weight loss, exercises on all six days, with low to moderate intensity, for 30 to 60 minutes is recommended. Longer exercise sessions increase the caloric expenditure.

The aerobics class, under the guidance of a trained instructor, gives optimum benefits. There is a group and a rhythmic beat. The atmosphere is safe, special flooring is provided, and mirrors help monitor your postures. Your instructor slowly increases your heart rate from resting to target intensity-level, in first 10 to 15 minutes, through a scientific warm-up session. This is maintained. Then you are in a training zone for the next 30 to 40 minutes. After which, your instructor slowly brings down the training and starts conditioning exercises for major muscle groups. Stretches are incorporated to drain the toxins formed during the exercises. Lastly, your heart rate is slowly lowered, by changing the tempo of music. If a relaxation session for 1 to 3 minutes is incorporated, it makes sure that the blood supply is again diverted to the vital organs, by maintaining the bell curve from the beginning to the last minute of the exercise. This whole session gives you a feeling of exhilaration. Group activity improves motivation through cross discussions. You feel you are not alone and the spirit of competition may help you adhere to the exercise routine well.

Warm-up: The purpose of a warm-up is to mobilize the joints and muscle groups. It prepares the body for vigorous exercises and minimizes the risk of injury. A warm-up consists of rhythmic limbering exercise that incorporates the use of joints and large muscle groups; static stretches are performed at a smooth and moderate rate. Stretches help prepare the body for more vigorous exercises by increasing the range of motion of joints to raise the temperature and heart rate. The warm-up helps minimize the risk of injury and maximize neuromuscular function. The duration of the warm-up should be 10 to 12 minutes with a music tempo of 110 to 120 bpm and static stretches for 2–3 minutes.

Benefits of Warm-Up

- Prepares the body for exercise in recommended intensity

- Increases flexibility of muscles, tendons and ligaments

- Increases core body temperature

- Increases heart rate and blood circulation to the muscles

- Increases lubrication of joints

- Prevents injuries, strain and muscle tears

- Warmer muscles produce faster and forceful contractions

- Reduces post-exercise soreness, increases overall flexibility by increasing the range of movements of the joints

- Mentally and physically mobilizes the individual and prepares him or her physiologically for activity

- Improves kinesthetic awareness

Special Dos and Don'ts

- Do rhythmic warm-up and stretches of the lower back.

- Do not do ballistic movements.

- Avoid overstretching of any ligament, tendon or lower back.

After warm-up, do an aerobic workout for 35 to 45 minutes. This portion should resemble a 'bell curve,' which means you should start slowly and gradually increase the intensity and range of movement. Then slowly bring it down during the cool-down session. You have to take care that prolonged continuous movements of large muscle groups are monitored.

Post-Aerobic Cool Down

This consists of 2–3 minutes of moderate slow-paced rhythmic movements for the upper and lower body, to enable the muscles of extremities to pump the blood back to the heart and the brain. Abrupt cessation could lead to light-headedness, dizziness or fainting. It is recommended that you hold the stretch for a minimum period of 10–20 seconds.

Walking

A very simple aerobic exercise that anybody can do anywhere is walking. It is the most natural, easiest, safest and least-expensive form of aerobic exercise. Do some warm-up exercises, like marching, before walking. Incorporate stretches and hand movements during warm-up. Monitor the heart rate and then start walking. You should cover at least 1 km in 9–10 minutes. Keep your spine in its natural curve. Continue it for at least 60 minutes. Monitor and make sure your intensity is in 70% of training zone. Walk longer steps and swing the arms back and forth. If you will walk for 1 hour with this intensity and cover a minimum of 6–7 km, then you will burn 300–400 calories per session.

Avoid Running

Walking is the best activity to start a conditioning program. Inactive people should start a 1-km walk first and then increase the time by five minutes every day. Light hand-weight and backpack help increase the intensity.

Use good sport shoes. They should be light in weight, flexible to take the shape of your feet and have good cushioning.

Avoid hard tar road. A jogging track is preferable. Avoid chatting while walking. As we discussed earlier, walking helps burn calories. It also helps in stress management and lowering cholesterol levels.

A word of caution: **Walking is not a complete exercise even though is a good exercise.**

Walking in Water

Walking in water at chest-deep level is also an excellent exercise for people with back and leg problems. The resistance from water adds intensity to the exercises.

Benefits of Aerobic Exercises

- *The heart becomes stronger and pumps more blood in single contraction. When you make your heart work in the training zone for 35 minutes, the heart muscle becomes stronger and improves the function of the cardiac output.*

- *Resting heart rate is reduced.*

- *The heart has to beat fewer number of times for the same cardiac output, which means its longevity increases.*

- *The capacity of your lungs increases.*

- *Maximum number of alveoli (air sacks) get utilized to supply the increased demand of oxygen to your muscle cells to produce more energy required to continue the activity.*

- *Elasticity of blood vessels increases due to additional work, as they perform rhythmically.*

- *Basal metabolism rate, that is the capacity of the body to burn calories, increases.*

- *Actually, calories from fats are utilized and this helps lose fats.*

- *Capillarization (number of capillaries} increases and forms a dense network of capillaries of the heart muscles as well as all the working muscles.*

- *This reduces the risk of ischemic heart diseases i.e. diseases of the heart due to loss of blood supply.*

- *Aerobic exercises are helpful in hypertension, diabetes, heart disease, anxiety, depression and obesity. The management of these diseases should incorporate aerobic exercises.*

- *These exercises increase good HDL cholesterol.*

- *They decrease bad LDL cholesterol and total cholesterol.*

- *They help in maintaining the recommended body composition.*

- *They help reducing the risk of osteoporosis.*

- *They control asthma and adult onset diabetes.*

- *They promote weight loss.*

- *They help manage stress.*

- *These exercises improve postural problems.*

- *They improve balance, agility, flexibility and strength.*

- *They improve the sense of wellbeing.*

- *They improve one's confidence.*

Obese people should avoid hiking, jogging, high-impact activities and skipping strictly. They should choose low-impact activities like swimming, water aerobics and cycling.

Swimming

Swimming uses many of the major muscle groups in the body. The risk of injuries is low. To benefit from the full intensity, like in ground exercises, avoid gliding strokes. Forward crawl is recommended.

The intensity must be enough to utilize more calories. In order to match the temperature after coming out of the water, one feels very hungry and wants to consume more food. Make sure you are not consuming more food than needed. Otherwise, negative energy balance will not be created. The excessive body fat makes the body more buoyant and the tendency is to float along often. This helps reduce stress but it does not increase calorie expenditure. To aid weight loss, walking or jogging in waist-deep water is better for overweight people who cannot walk or jog on the ground. Calorie expenditure per hour is comparatively lesser in swimming than compared to jogging for an hour.

Cycling

Cycling provides cardio-respiratory endurance, muscular strength and endurance in lower extremities. It does not raise the heart rate, as fast as other aerobic exercises do, because, in cycling, only the thigh muscles are used. However, by increasing the duration of cycling, one can achieve the same output. Of course, it puts less stress on muscles and joints compared to jogging. Therefore, cycling is recommended to people who cannot walk or jog.

The height of the bicycle should be adjusted so that the legs are almost completely extended when they are placed on the pedals. The body should not sway from side to side as the person rides the bicycle. The bike tension should be set at a moderate level to be able to ride at 60 to 100 revolutions per minute.

You have to wear appropriate clothes and shoes. Special clothing for cycling is not required. For great comfort, some extra padding can be sewn into the crotch areas. An experienced cyclist often wears special shoes—cleats that snap onto the pedal.

In order to make the weight-loss program injury-free and safe, high-intensity and high-impact activities are usually considered. Although they burn more calories, they are avoided by the weight-loss population. Injuries to muscles and joints are very common in overweight individuals who engage in aerobic exercises.

To start a scientific regimen of exercise for your weight loss, you have to become mobile first. Then slowly, you can increase the physical activity.

Follow the tips given below to design a safe and effective workout.

- Warm-up exercises: Stationary bike, slow walk or marching with low intensity with simple hand movements for 10–20 minutes

- Strength training: Involve all major muscle groups with low resistance and more repetitions. Perform 12 exercises in two sets.

- Body conditioning exercises for all muscle groups

- Cooling-down stretches: Flexibility training for all muscle groups

When your fitness increases, you can do strength training on alternate days with an intensity of 12–15 repetitions. You will get strength and endurance and will be able to increase the lean body weight. Practice strength training for three alternate days a week, followed by flexibility training.

On the remaining alternate three days of the week, aerobic workout with intensity of 40–60% of the target zone for 35–40 minutes is recommended. Perform warm-up and cool-down exercises during every session.

As your fitness increases, you overload your body and increase all the components of fitness viz. strength, endurance, cardio-respiratory endurance and flexibility. This will help improve your body composition, BMR, AMR, and total calorie expenditure during the day. You will convert your body into a machine that can utilize calories at a better rate than before or with a calorie-burning precision like that of an athlete.

Flexibility Training

Flexibility is one of the important components of fitness. Flexibility means the capacity of muscles and connective tissues i.e. tendons and ligaments, to get stretched to their maximum range. If we cannot stretch them to their maximum range, the range of motion of the joint will be reduced. This may lead to injury, when we try to reach that particular range, when required in our day-to-day activity.

As we decrease physical activity, muscles lose their elasticity and tendons and ligaments tighten up and shorten. Aging also reduces extensibility of soft tissues. This results in decreased flexibility.

Generally, flexibility exercises are performed after an aerobic workout or after proper warm-up.

If muscles are not warmed up before stretching, the range of movement will get reduced by 20%.

The overload and specificity of training principles should be applied for development of muscular flexibility. To improve the total range of motion i.e. flexibility, the muscles surrounding the joints have to be stretched progressively beyond their accustomed length.

Mode

- Ballistic stretching

- Slow sustained stretching

- Proprioceptive neuromuscular facilitation stretching. Each type has certain benefits.

- Ballistic or dynamic stretching provides the necessary force to lengthen the muscles. Such type of stretching is to be avoided in a weight-loss program as it may cause soreness, injury, overstretching of ligaments, subluxations and dislocations.

- Slow and sustained stretching: This type causes the muscles to relax, thereby achieving greater length. It causes little pain and has a low risk of injury. This type should be used by the weight-loss population.

- Proprioceptive neuromuscular facilitation: This technique is based on the 'contract and relax' principle. Here we require the assistance of a trainer.

- The initial force is provided by the assistant. He pushes slowly in the direction of the desired stretch. At the initial stage, the desired range is not achieved.

- The individual then applies force in the direction opposite to the assistant through isometric contraction.

- This leads to relaxation of muscles. Then the assistant increases the stretch slowly to a greater range.

- Isometric contraction is repeated for another 4–5 seconds, following which the muscle relaxes. This increases the degree of stretch. The final stage is held for 10–30 seconds.

Intensity

The intensity should be only to a point of mild discomfort. Excessive pain is to be avoided. All stretches should be done slightly below the pain threshold. At this point, you should try to relax the muscle under stretch as much as possible. You may take the help of long breathing techniques. Each stretch should be done for four times, holding the final position for 10–30 seconds. As the flexibility increases, the time of holding can be increased.

Frequency

We have to incorporate stretches at the end of the warm-up session. This will help eliminate toxins like lactic acid, which were formed in the exercises done earlier in the day. It will also help give the full range of motion throughout the workout. Also, stretches should be incorporated in the cool-down phase. This helps to improve the overall flexibility.

For attaining more flexibility, give your body proper time.

Yogasana improves the flexibility of joints. Conversely, if you have good flexibility, you can do yogasana properly. While yoga is useful for flexibility and is a good exercise of body as well as mind, **pranayama** helps consume more oxygen, which enhances metabolism to some extent, though with limitations.

Meditation is the best mode of relaxation. Many medical conditions, like lower back pain, neck pain, knee pain, joint pain and shoulder pain are corrected by proper flexibility training of the muscles surrounding the joints. Physical inactivity, poor postural habits and body mechanics, and excessive weight are the reasons for these conditions. To treat these conditions, you have to be physically active, improve your postural habits and lose the excessive weight. (Refer to the pyramid at the end of this chapter.)

Tips to Enhance Adherence to Exercise

You can take many days to introduce this new aspect of exercise in your healthy lifestyle. Many times, you are enthusiastic to start the program. You buy an alarm clock, a new pair of shoes and a track suit and set a big goal to start a vigorous exercise regimen. But you get tired due to your long-term physical inactivity. You may feel sick and you tend to drop out. To avoid this, you have to chalk a successful plan. You must enjoy your workout. The logic is simple. If you enjoy what you do, you will continue to do it.

For the first few weeks, you will find it difficult but remember, where there is a will there is a way. Once you begin to see the positive changes, it will not be so difficult. Soon you will make exercise a habit. This will be deeply satisfying and bring a sense of accomplishment. The following suggestions will help you accept the change in your lifestyle and adhere to it as a lifetime exercise program.

- *Set aside a regular time for exercise. If you do not find time, plan ahead. It is a lot easier to skip exercise but tougher to stick to it. Hold your exercise hour 'sacred.' Give exercise the same priority you would give to an important task.*

- *Try to be physically active throughout the day. Take the stairs instead of the elevator. Walk the dog and ride the stationary bike while watching TV.*

- *Select the exercise of your choice, so that it is enjoyable.*

- *Try to join a health club where somebody monitors your exercise and modifies it, as per your physical fitness status, requirement and progress. In case you absent yourself, there should be somebody who asks you about it. In case of pain, you need someone to suggest alternatives. Don't be afraid to try a new activity, even if it means learning new skills.*

- *Wear proper clothing and use appropriate equipment for exercise. A poor pair of shoes, for instance, can make you more prone to injury and may discourage you from the beginning.*

- *Find a friend or a group to exercise with you. Social interaction will make exercise more fulfilling. Besides, it is harder to skip if somebody is waiting for you.*

- *Set short goals and share them with others. Quitting is tougher when someone knows what you are trying to accomplish. When you achieve a targeted goal, reward yourself with new T-shirt.*

- *Listen to your body. Over-exercising may lead to chronic fatigue and injuries. Enjoy the exercise.*

- *Try to add variety in your workout.*

- *Exercise with music. The tempo of music adds vigor to the workout.*

- *Keep a regular record of your activities to monitor your progress.*

- *Conduct periodic assessments to notice progress. Higher fitness is a reward in itself.*

- *If you experience unusual discomfort or pain, do not ignore it. Pains and aches are indications of potential injuries. Do not aggravate the injury. Rest the part and find out an alternative. If the leg is injured, work the upper body or midsection. Only if it is required, take full rest.*

- *In case of health problems, consult a physician.*

- *Safety is the first priority.*

- *Remember, fitness is not a quick-fix medicine. Fitness takes time and dedication and only those who are committed and persistent will reap the rewards.*

- *Set realistic goals. (Refer to the chapter on setting goals.)*

- *In case you are out of station, try to find a hotel with a health club or a swimming pool.*

- *The simple solution is to walk. Morning hours are totally yours. Try to enjoy nature at various places. A one-hour brisk walk with conditioning exercises will give you good calorie output.*

While doing weight-loss, do not skip any session of the workout, for any reason. It affects the weight loss during that week. Then you are compelled to eat less as you have missed the workout. Then you feel hungry and it becomes difficult for you to adhere to the diet program. This affects your psyche to adhere to a total change. You may eat something wrong, feel guilty, compensate for it the next day, do more and get more demotivated. The vicious circle would definitely start.

Even if you eat something you should not, do not try to burn the extra calories on the same day by doing more exercise. You should not have a punishing attitude. Try to be disciplined from the next day. Exercise is for health. It is not a punishment or compensation for what you have eaten wrongly.

Use this simple logic. If you consume 600 calories more than your daily plan by having 3–4 ice cream scoops, then to burning 600 calories, you need to walk for two additional hours to cover another 12 km, at a speed of 6 kms per hour, which is not possible in your daily routine. So, do not develop such a grueling attitude of compensation. Instead, try to be disciplined and determined throughout your whole program.

Note down the positive and negative changes that occur in your mind, after accepting the new change of incorporating exercise in your routine. Note down the graph of progress.

After three months, you will realize that you have a good strong body. You are lifting almost double weights during every exercise. Your endurance has gone up and you are doing more repetitions, more sit-ups and push-ups, which you were hardly able to do earlier. Your flexibility has improved you and you can bend easily while lacing your shoes, without any pain.

Your stamina has reached the higher level. You can climb up the staircase without any break and without huffing and puffing. Your measurements are reducing. Your mirror image is reminding you of your college days. You feel you are resembling your favorite model, hero or sportsperson, someone who is fit.

Feel proud. Feel great that you have conquered a new milestone on the path toward a slim, healthy and fit body, by making exercise a part and parcel of your day-to-day life.

Exercise Chart

1 Little, 2 Medium, 3 Good, 4 Better, 5 Excellent

Type	Kcal/hr.	S	E	F	CRE
Gym	400	5	5	4	3
Aerobics	400	3	4	4	5
Walk (6 km/hr)	300	2	3	2	4
Jogging (9 km/hr)	500	4	3	2	5
Cycle (8 km/hr)	250	3	3	2	3
Cycle (I9 km/hr)	400	4	3	2	5
Swimming					
(Fast, nonstop)	500	4	4	3	5

S	–	**Strength**
E	–	**Endurance**
F	–	**Flexibility**
CRE	–	**Cardio-respiratory endurance**

Chapter 9

Basics of Nutrition and Balanced Diet for Weight Loss

Introduction

A balanced and nutritious diet is essential for weight control. This chapter will provide you information on the basics of nutrition and the requirements for a well-balanced diet for overall good health and to achieve and maintain a healthy weight.

Variety and moderation are the keys to a healthy diet. You have to eliminate junk from your diet and plan a low-cal but nutritious menu, which will help you achieve the targeted weight.

In this chapter, a food pyramid with low-cal Indian food is given along with minute details such as serving size. Special emphasis is given on detailed information of fibers, cholesterol, antioxidants and water with low-cal sources of protective foods such as vitamins and minerals. This information will help you to know how to increase your immunity to fight certain chronic disorders like cancer and cholesterol. Eat healthy, get healthy. After all, you are what you eat!

Food is the fuel that keeps the body alive. The pleasures of a meal are among the joys of life. Proper nutrition through this joy is the only way toward good health and wellbeing. Eating for health does not prohibit the pleasure of eating. We have to reorganize our food habits, which will provide nutrition. This means a diet that supplies all essential nutrients for normal tissue growth, repair and maintenance and enough substrates to produce the energy required to perform day-to-day work, physical activity and relaxation, with optimum efficiency.

Lack of awareness about balanced diet and nutrition often plays a crucial role in development and progression of diseases. For instance, a diet high in saturated fats and cholesterol increases the risk of atherosclerosis (thickening of blood vessels) and coronary heart diseases. High salt intake may lead to hypertension (blood pressure that is more than normal). Most of the cancers are diet related. Diabetes mellitus, osteoporosis and obesity are also associated with faulty nutrition.

You must know some basics of nutrition before planning your diet for health, wellbeing and weight reduction in a scientific way.

Essential Nutrients

The essential nutrients the human body requires are carbohydrates, fats, proteins, vitamins, minerals and water.

- **Carbohydrates:** This group is a major source of calories that the body uses to provide energy for work, cell maintenance and heat. They help regulate fat and metabolize protein. One gram of carbohydrate provides 4 kcal of energy.

The major sources of carbohydrates are sugar, jaggery, honey, cereals, grains, fruits, vegetables, pulses, milk and dairy products.

Carbohydrates are divided into simple carbohydrates and complex carbohydrates.

Simple carbohydrates: Sugar, jaggery, honey, alcohol, candy and soda have little nutritive value. They get absorbed in the blood immediately and their TEF is extremely less.

Facts about honey

Honey is a unique carbohydrate. It begins as nectar in the flower and is harvested by the honey bee and transported to a hive. At this point, it is sucrose with enzyme invertase. In the honeycomb, it is converted into glucose and fructose. After prolonged evaporation, the concentrated product is stored in a sealed cell of honeycomb. The typical final composition of honey is glucose 34%, fructose 41%, sucrose 2.4% and water 18.3%.

Most of the honey available in the market has been processed to a temperature of 150–160 °C to prevent crystallization and yeast fermentation that may occur during storage. Organic honey is unprocessed raw honey.

The low temperatures used in the processing of honey are not sufficient to destroy the spores of clostridium botulism. These spores sometimes favor spore germination and toxin formation in the digestive system of very young infants and causes infant botulism. It is, therefore, not advisable to feed honey to an infant till he or she reaches the age of one year.

The popular belief is that, honey along with lemon water, is helpful to reduce weight. However, it provides 6.4 kcal per gram, which is greater than that the energy provided by one gram of sugar, which is 4 kcal. Honey contains some vitamins and minerals, which are not available in sugar. However, the amount is not up to the mark in terms of daily needs. It seems honey is neither helpful in lowering weight nor does it provide extraordinary nutrients. It should not to consumed by children till the age of one year, diabetics and obese people.

Complex carbohydrates: Linking of simple carbohydrates lead to formation of complex carbohydrates or starches. Complex carbohydrates provide many valuable nutrients and they are also an excellent source of fiber (roughage).

After digestion, complex carbohydrates get converted into simple carbohydrates i.e. glucose, fructose, maltose and lactose, which get absorbed into the blood and get utilized by the body as an immediate source of energy. Additional glucose is converted into glycogen and is stored in muscles and liver. When a surge of energy is needed, the enzymes in the muscles and liver break down glycogen and make glucose readily available for energy transformation.

Carbohydrates are the body's best source of energy. They provide protein-sparing action. If one does not consume carbohydrates in the required amount, then proteins have to perform the function of energy production. However, they are considerably more expensive, both in cost and in the amount of energy required for metabolism. Sufficient intake of carbohydrates spares the proteins from being involved in energy formation.

A nutritious diet must contain 60% of carbohydrate, preferably the complex kind.

Fiber: Fiber is a form of complex carbohydrate. Dietary fiber is present mainly in plant leaves, skins, roots and seeds. Processing and refining food remove almost all the natural fiber in foods. But the role of fiber in diet is extremely important. Fiber is a rich source of vitamins and minerals. When you consume fibrous foods, you automatically get the requisite vitamins and minerals.

Fibers are classified into two groups: soluble fiber that can dissolve in water and form a gel-like substance that encloses the food particle. This property allows soluble fiber to bind and excrete fats from the body. Soluble fibers are composed of pectin and guar gums. Soluble fiber has been proven as a reason for the decrease in blood cholesterol and blood sugar levels. It decreases the risk of cardiovascular diseases. Increased fiber intake lowers the risk of heart diseases because saturated fats often take the place of fiber in diet, which increases the absorption and formation of cholesterol. The sensitivity of insulin also seems to improve because of a fiber-rich diet, which helps in controlling diabetes and obesity. Soluble fibers are found primarily in oats, fruits, barley and legumes.

The other type of fiber is insoluble fiber. Insoluble fiber cannot dissolve in water and the body cannot digest it. This fiber is important as it binds water, resulting in softer, bulkier stools that increase peristalsis i.e. movement of the intestines, the involuntary contraction of the muscles of the intestinal walls, forcing the stools outward and allowing food residues to pass through the intestinal track more quickly. Speeding up of the passage of food through the intestines seems to lower the risk of colon cancer by avoiding contact with cancer-causing agents, with the walls of the intestine for a longer time. Also, insoluble fibers bind with cancer-causing substances, thus lessening their potency. Insoluble fiber also decreases the risk of diverticulitis, piles (hemorrhoids), gall bladder disease, obesity and constipation. Sources of insoluble fibers are vegetables, fruit skins, wheat, cereals and bran.

High-fiber food gets swollen in the stomach. This leads to mechanical contact of food with the walls of the stomach. This gives signals of satiety to the brain, providing a feeling of fullness. A low-calorie diet, followed by consumption of fiber-rich-food, provides the full satisfaction of having eaten a full meal. Fiber also lingers in the stomach, helping one feel full for a longer duration.

Caution should be taken to introduce fiber-rich food gradually to avoid stomach upset, bloating, flatulence and diarrhea. It is also important to drink lots of water when adding fiber to the diet because fiber acts like a sponge and attracts water. The recommended amount of fiber is 25 to 35 grams per day. Adding more than 35 grams of fiber may interfere with the absorption of some essential minerals.

Tips to Increase Fiber in Diet

- Eat more vegetables, either raw or steamed, before every meal. Two bowls of salads before every meal, i.e. breakfast, lunch and dinner, is advisable (total 6 bowls a day).

- Eat salads that include a wide variety of seasonal vegetables in varied colors.

- Eat fruit with skin.

- Use whole wheat flour. Do not sieve it.

- Eat finger millet, puffed grains, legumes and pulses with skin. Dishes like various types of breads should be made using green leafy vegetables. Add salads while preparing any salty, spicy, low-cal porridge and thick soups.

- Use vegetables in sandwiches. Eat green and red pepper stripes, diced carrots, sliced cucumber, red cabbage and onion with brown bread.

- Prepare rolls of whole grain breads using stuffing of broccoli, cauliflower, mushroom, sliced carrots and leafy vegetables.

- Prepare cutlets using steamed vegetables of various colors. Bind them with wheat flour with wheat bran.

- Use lots of vegetables in all preparations mixed with finely chopped salads and dressed with lime juice and spices.

- Try out unfamiliar fruits and vegetables, which are juicy, watery and rich in fibers.

- Drink plenty of water, minimum 10–12 glasses of water per day.

Fats

Fats or lipids are the most concentrated sources of energy. Each gram of fat supplies 9 kcal of energy. Fats are a part of the cell structure. Fats are used as stored energy and as an insulator to preserve body heat.

The fat depots work as shock absorbers to protect vital organs. Fats supply essential fatty acids and carry fat-soluble vitamins (A, D, E and K). The main sources of fats are oil, butter, ghee, red meat or animal fats, oil seeds, palm oil and ghee. Fats are classified as simple fats, compound fats and derived fats.

Simple fats consist of glyceride molecule, linked with one, two or three units of fatty acids. According to the number of fatty acids attached to them, simple fats are divided into monoglycerides (one fatty acid), diglyceride (two fatty acids) and triglycerides (three fatty acids). More than 90% of the weight of fats in food and 95% of the weight of stored fat in the human body are in the form of triglycerides.

Fatty acids are further classified as saturated and unsaturated, based on the extent of saturation. Unsaturated fatty acids are further classified as polyunsaturated and monounsaturated. Saturated fats are mainly of animal origin. Unsaturated fats are generally found in plant products.

In saturated fats, the carbon atoms are fully saturated with hydrogen; only single bonds link the carbon atoms to the chain. Red meat, lard, whole milk, cream, butter, cheese, ice cream, hydrogenated oil (they are saturated by processing), coconut oil and palm oil are examples of saturated fats. In unsaturated fats, there is a double bond between the unsaturated carbons and monounsaturated fatty acids (MUFA have only one double bond along the chain.) Corn, cottonseed, safflower, walnut, sunflower and soyabean are high in polyunsaturated fatty acids.

Saturated fats tend to be solids that typically do not melt at room temperature, while unsaturated fats are usually liquid at room temperature. Coconut and palm oil are exceptions to this rule. Even though they are high in saturated fats, they are liquid at room temperature. In general, saturated fats raise the blood cholesterol level, whereas polyunsaturated and monounsaturated fats lower the blood cholesterol.

Compound fats are a combination of simple fats and other chemicals. Examples are phospholipids, glucolipids and lipoproteins.

Derived fats combine simple and compound fats. E.g. sterols. Although sterol contains no fatty acids, they are considered lipids because they do not dissolve in water. The most-often mentioned sterol is cholesterol, which is found in many foods or can be manufactured from saturated fats.

Cholesterol: Cholesterol is a complex waxy substance. It is an essential component of the walls of body cells. It is also used to make vitamin D, hormones, bile acids and nerve tissue. It is carried around the body in the blood stream by lipoproteins (proteins to which lipids or fats are attached). High levels of cholesterol increase the chances of having a heart attack. Only about 15% of the total cholesterol comes from diet, the remaining is made in the liver continuously. As a result, some of the excess dietary cholesterol may get deposited in the blood vessels and the rest is eliminated.

Cholesterol is transported primarily in the form of high-density lipoprotein (HDL). When HDL comes in contact with cholesterol-filled cells, the protein molecules in the coating of HDL get attached to the cholesterol-filled cells and take their cholesterol. On the other hand, low-density lipoprotein (LDL) releases cholesterol. This released cholesterol may penetrate the lining of the arteries and speed up the process of atherosclerosis. HDL cholesterol is good cholesterol and offers some protection against heart diseases. Women have higher levels of HDL as estrogen tends to raise HDL.

Higher the intensity of aerobic exercise, higher is the level of HDL cholesterol. Saturated fats raise cholesterol levels more than anything in the diet. Every person has a different tendency to have different levels of cholesterol even though they consume the same amount of saturated fats. Unsaturated cannot be converted to cholesterol.

Lowering LDL Cholesterol

If LDL cholesterol or bad cholesterol is higher than ideal, it can be lowered by losing body fat, manipulating diet, taking medication and participating in a regular aerobic exercise.

Medication acts by decreasing the absorption of cholesterol in the intestines or by blocking cholesterol formation by the cells. These drugs can cause muscle and joint pain and affect lever enzyme level. It is better to lower the LDL cholesterol by changing the lifestyle. Low-fat, low saturated fat, low cholesterol and high-fiber diet is recommended in a changed lifestyle. Saturated fat should be replaced by monounsaturated and polyunsaturated fats. Polyunsaturated fats tend to decrease LDL cholesterol. Exercise is also very important. Diet and exercise are the only most effective combination to lower LDL cholesterol.

An intake with 30 grams fiber per day, total fat less than 20% of the total calorie intake, consumption of as less saturated fats as possible and an average cholesterol consumption of less than 30 mg per day are the dietary recommendations. Soluble fiber dissolves in water, forms a gel-like substance, and encloses food particles. This helps bind and excrete the fats from the body. Such a type of diet is practically difficult to follow. But such a diet with aerobic exercise is useful to lower 23% of cholesterol in three weeks. For weight reduction, these recommendations can be followed. For maintenance of lower level, a diet with 30% fat with 10% saturated fats and 300 mg cholesterol will be helpful. A low-fat diet also leads to lower HDL levels and increased triglycerides. In such a case, monounsaturated and polyunsaturated fats are to be added to the diet by removing saturated fats. Stanol ester, a plant derived-compound, lowers LDL cholesterol by 14%.

How to Lower LDL Cholesterol Level

- *Consume 25 to 30 grams of fiber with minimum 10 grams of soluble fiber (oats, fruits, barley, legumes).*

- *Consume 25 grams of soy protein every day.*

- *Avoid organ meat and red meat.*

- *Avoid commercially baked foods.*

- *Avoid foods containing trans-fatty acids, hydrogenated fats and partially hydrogenated oil.*

- *Drink low-fat milk and milk products.*

- *Eat fish instead of red meat.*

- *Bake, boil, grill, poach or steam food instead of frying.*

- *Cooked meat when refrigerated brings fats to th4e top. They need to be removed before eating.*

- *Avoid fatty sauces made with butter, cream and cheese.*

- *Avoid coconut oil, palm oil, vanaspati, palm ghee and butter.*

- *Avoid egg yellow.*

- *Maintain recommended body weight.*

- *Remember the 3Fs – fiber-rich, fat-free, fish.*

- *A diet with these 3 Fs fights will lower LDL.*

Triglycerides

Triglycerides or free fatty acids, in combination with cholesterol, speed up the formation of plaque. Very low-density lipoprotein (VLDL) and chylomicron carry triglycerides in the blood stream.

These fatty acids are found in poultry skin, red meats, shellfish but they are manufactured in the liver from refined sugars, starches and alcohol. A high intake of alcohol, sugars, starches and honey significantly raises triglyceride levels. Aerobic exercise, weight reduction and avoiding the above-mentioned foods help reduce triglycerides.

Triglycerides and cholesterol are discussed here in detail, for the much-needed awareness about their role and function and how to control their use to prevent coronary heart diseases and obesity.

Type	Dietary fat	Dietary cholesterol mg/tbsp	% Saturated fats	% Poly unsaturated fats	% Mono unsaturated fats
M	Canola oil	0	6	32	62
P	Safflower oil	0	10	77	13
P	Sunflower oil	0	11	69	20
P	Corn oil	0	13	62	25
M	Olive oil	0	14	9	77

continue…

M	Peanut oil	0	18	33	49
P	Soyabean oil	0	15	61	24
S	Chicken fat	11	31	22	47
S	Beef fat	14	52	4	44
S	Butter	33	66	4	30

M – Monosaturated, P – Polyunsaturated S – Saturated

Essential Fatty Acids

Although there is a link between a high-fat diet, obesity and heart disease, there should not be fear of fat. Some essential fatty acids are vital for proper functioning, growth and maintenance of body. They are a group of polyunsaturated fats. Linoleic and linolenic are two of the essential fatty acids required in the diet. They can be transformed to other essential fatty acids by our body. Sunflower oil, corn oil, peanut, breast milk, soybean/oil seed oil, fish liver oil and fish are the sources of essential fatty acids.

Essential fatty acids are useful in preventing blood clotting, reduction of cholesterol production, boosting of insulin activity, and enhancement of immune activity (to fight asthma, allergies and arthritis). Antioxidants are required to be consumed in sufficient quantity for good activity of essential fatty acids. EPA (*eicosapentaenoic* acid) and DHA (docosahexanoic acid) are known as omega 3 fatty acids. They are found in fish oil and linseed oil. These fatty acids prevent the aggregation of blood platelets to form clots. They allow the cells to pass through the smallest blood vessels capillaries. In this way, EPA and DHA can help prevent ischemic heart diseases (heart diseases caused when blood supply to the heart muscle is stopped partially or totally), as they prevent sticking of the blood cells in the tiny vessels and causing oxygen deficiency to the heart tissue.

Nowadays, supplements containing GLA, EPA and DHA are available in the market. They get easily utilized in the body. Along with antioxidants (vitamin C, beta carotene, vitamin E and selenium), these supplements are extremely useful in many disorders.

Proteins

The main function of protein is to build and repair tissue, including muscles, blood, internal organs, skin, hair, nails and bones. They are a part of hormones, enzymes and antibodies and help maintain a normal balance of body fluids. Proteins can also be used as a source of energy but only if carbohydrates are not available. 1 gram of protein provides 4 kcal of energy. The primary sources of proteins are lean meat, skinless chicken, white fish, eggs, milk, milk products, legumes, pulses, some grains, soybean.

Proteins are composed of amino acids containing nitrogen, carbon, hydrogen and oxygen. Nine out of 20 amino acids are called essential amino acids, as the body cannot produce them. The other 11 non-essential amino acids can be manufactured in the body if food protein in the diet provides enough nitrogen. For normal function of the body, all amino acids must be present at the same time.

Two glasses of skimmed milk and 200 grams of lean meat, in terms of poultry or fish, meet the daily protein requirement. However, protein deficiency could be a concern in some vegetarian diets. Vegetarians must be careful to eat foods that provide a balanced distribution of essential amino acids such as grains and legumes.

Grains and cereals are low in amino acids; lysine and legumes lack methionine (one of the non-essential amino acids). Combining food from these two groups (*idli* and *sambhar, dal* and *chawal, roti* and legumes, rice and soybean) will help compensate for each other. Combining both groups in the same meal will be helpful than taking them separately at various times.

Grains	+	nuts and seeds
Grains	+	legumes
Grains	+	milk products
Nuts and seeds	+	legumes
Milk products	+	legumes

The combinations suggested above can give complete protein.

Grains: Brown rice, whole wheat and oats (fiber-rich grains)

Legumes: Soybean, *moong, masoor (red grams), matki (small grams), toor (yellow gram), kuleeth* (low-calorie legumes)

Seeds and Nuts: They are sources of fat too. When included in the diet, balancing of calories is to be taken into consideration.

Dairy Products: Skimmed milk, cow's milk without cream, curds, buttermilk

A non-vegetarian diet provides complete proteins but if it is consumed without care then it provides lots of fats and calories and encourages weight gain. There are some high-protein fad diets, which are used to lose the weight. The serious consequences of these are increased ketone bodies, potassium and calcium depletion, muscle weakness and a possible kidney problem.

Out of the total calories consumed, 20% of them must be contributed by proteins, says the principle of balanced diet. Non-vegetarian proteins should be consumed by eliminating fats from them. Red meat is to be avoided. Chicken without skin, white fish and egg whites are to be included in the diet to avoid saturated fats and cholesterol.

Vitamins

Vitamins are vital amines essential to life. They play a key role in all body activities like energy production, growth, maintenance and repair. They are needed in small amounts. They must be obtained from the diet as the body cannot manufacture them. Vitamins perform various functions as antioxidants (A, C, E), co-enzymes (B complex) and hormones (D).

Based on their solubility, vitamins are divided into two categories.

Water-soluble   B and C

Fat-soluble   A, D, E, K

If the diet is balanced, containing the recommended servings from the five-food groups, then, as few as 1,200 calories per day can fulfill the nutrient requirements of the body. Vitamins in the recommended dietary allowance through natural sources are to be taken preferably. One should avoid vitamin supplements unless they are advised by the physician.

Minerals

Regulation of heart beat, formation of hemoglobin in the blood for transportation of oxygen to every cell, building of bones and teeth and muscle contraction are the important functions in the body. They are possible because of various minerals in our daily diet. Minerals are inorganic substances and are constituents of all cells, especially in the hard parts. They are crucial in maintaining water balance and acid base balance. They are essential components of respiratory pigments and enzyme system. Major minerals like calcium, phosphorous, sodium chloride and magnesium are required in amounts greater than 100 mg every day. Whereas minor minerals are required in smaller amount. They include iron, zinc, copper and iodine etc. Various sources and functions are included in the following table.

Vitamins Chart

Vitamin	U.S. RDA	Best sources	Functions
A (carotene)	5,000 IU/day	Yellow or orange fruits and vegetables, green leafy vegetable, fortified oatmeal liver, dairy products	Formation and maintenance of skin, hair and mucous membranes; helps you see in dim light; bone and tooth growth
B1 (thiamine)	1.5 mg/day	Fortified cereals, millets, rice, pasta whole grains, liver	Helps body release energy from carbohydrates during metabolism; growth and muscle tone
B2 (riboflavin)	1.7 mg/day	Whole grains, green leafy vegetables, organ meats milk and eggs,	Helps body release energy from protein, fat and carbohydrates during metabolism
B6 pyridoxine	2 mg/day	Fish, poultry, lean meats bananas, dried beans, whole grains, avocado	Helps build body tissue; aids in metabolism of protein
B12	6	Meats, milk products, seafood	Aids cell development, functioning of the nervous system and the metabolism of protein fat
Biotin	0.3 mg/day	Cereal, grain products, yeast, legumes, liver	Involved in metabolism of protein, fats and carbohydrates
Folate (Folacin folic acid)	0.4 mg/day	Green leafy vegetables, organ meats, dried peas, beans and lentils	Aids in genetic material development; involved in red blood cell production
Niacin	20 mg/day	Meat, poultry, fish, enriched cereals, peanuts, potatoes, dairy products, eggs	Involved in carbohydrates, proteins and fat metabolism
Pantothenic acid	10 mg/day	Lean meats, whole grains, legumes, vegetables, fruits	Helps release energy from fats and carbohydrates
C (ascorbic acid)	60 mg/day	Citrus fruits, berries and vegetables, especially peppers	Essential for structure of bones, cartilage, muscle and blood vessels; helps maintain capillaries and gums; aids in absorption of iron.
D	400 IU/day	Fortified milk, sunlight, fish, eggs, butter, fortified margarine	Aids in bone and tooth formation; helps maintain heart action and nervous system
E	30 IU/day	Fortified and multi-grain cereals, nuts, wheat germ vegetable oils, green leafy vegetables	Protects blood cells, body tissue and essential fatty acids from harmful destruction in the body
K	—	Green leafy vegetables, fruits, dairy and grain products	Essential for blood clotting function

Minerals Chart

Calcium	1000 mg/day	Milk and milk products	For strong bones, teeth, muscle tissue; regulates heartbeat, muscle action and nerve function; aids blood clotting
Chromium	No RDA	Corn oil, dams, whole grain cereals, brewer's yeast	Glucose metabolism energy; increases effectiveness of insulin
Copper	2 mg/day	Oysters, nuts, organ, meats, legumes	Formation of red blood cells, bone growth and health; works with vitamin C to from elastin
Iodine	150 mg/day	Seafood, iodized salt	Component of hormone thyroxin, which controls metabolism
Iron mg/day	18 legumes	Meats, organ meat	Improves blood quality, hemoglobin formation; improves resistance to stress and disease
Magnesium	No RDA	Nuts, green vegetables whole grain	For acid/alkaline balance; important in metabolism of carbohydrates, minerals and sugar
Manganese	No RDA	Nuts, whole grains, vegetables, fruits	Enzyme activation; carbohydrates and fat production; sex hormone production; skeletal development
Phosphorus	1000 mg/day	Fish, meat, poultry, eggs, grains	Bone development, important in protein, fat and carbohydrate utilization.
Potassium	No RDA	Lean meat, vegetables, fruits	Fluid balance; controls activity of heart muscle, nervous system and kidneys
Selenium	50–20 mcg/ day RDA	Seafood, organ meat, lean meat, organs grains	Protects body tissue against oxidative damage from radiation pollution and normal metabolic processing
Zinc	15 mg/day	Lean meat, liver, eggs, seafood, whole grain	Involved in digestion and metabolism; important in development of reproductive system; aids in healing

Water

Next to oxygen, water is an extremely necessary and important nutrient to sustain life. It is the most abundant substance in the body accounting for 60–70% of the body's weight.

All tissues contain water in various amounts. It makes up 75% of muscle tissue and only 25% of fat tissue. The body weight of a lean person is comprised of a relatively high percentage of water. Conversely, the body weight of an individual with a high percentage of body fat is made up of a considerably low percentage of water.

Every cell relies on water to carry out all its activities. Thus, the body uses water for almost all its functions. Water transports nutrients to the cells and removes wastes from the cells. It also helps regulate the body temperature.

If enough water is not consumed, one feels fatigued and there is a faulty regulation of body temperature. This results in an increased risk of heat exhaustion and heat stroke. A less active person should drink eight glasses of water per day and a person engaged in moderate-to-strenuous activity should drink more water. Thirst should not be an indicator that your body needs water. By the time you feel thirsty, you will be on your way to dehydration. Water is the vehicle and the medium for all metabolic activities in the body like digestion, absorption, elimination of waste, building and rebuilding cells, and transporting nutrients.

The color of urine should always match the color of water. Dark urine is an indicator of dehydration.

Water is a major constituent of all foods but it is primarily found in liquid foods, fruits and vegetables. Plain water should not be substituted with tea, coffee and cold drinks. Adding sugar and salt in water increases the calorie value of the daily calorie input; 1 gram of salt may lead to the retention of 60 grams of water in the body.

In some disorders like high blood pressure, cardiac failure and urinary diseases, physiological conditions like premenstrual phase pregnancy and late nights, conditions like hypoproteinamia (less proteins) and hormonal imbalance, water gets retained in the body, showing edema i.e. swelling on the face, ankles, feet, thighs and hips. Drinking lots of water helps in diuresis (increase in urine production) and elimination of extra fluid. The benefits of drinking water have been discussed in an earlier chapter on energy.

One serving of carbohydrates (one out of the below mentioned choices): *1 roti, 1 chapati/Type of bread 1 idli/rice & gram Cake, 1 small dosa/pancake of rice & gram, 1 small uttappam pancake of rice & gram, 1 khakra/type of bread, 1 thepla/type of bread, 1 dhirde/type of bread, 1 bread slice. ½ bowl of 200 gm rice, ½ bowl of poha, ½ bowl of cooked daliya, ½ bowl of upma (spicy porridge), ½ bowl of oats ½ bowl ukad (porridge), 1 bowl of 200 gm. puffed grains*

One serving of vegetables
1 bowl cooked or raw vegetables

One serving of fruits
1 apple, 1 pear, 1 guava, 1 fig, 1 orange, 1 sweet lime, 1 pomegranate, 6 strawberries, 6 berries, 1 bowl papaya, 1 bowl musk melon, 1 bowl watermelon.

One serving of milk
1 cup of milk, 1 cup of curds, 1 glass buttermilk

One serving of dal
1 bowl thin dal, 1 bowl sprouts

One serving of eggs or meat
2 eggs white, 100 grams of chicken i.e. breast piece, 1 piece tuna fish

Fats, oils and sweets are to be consumed as less as possible. The top of the pyramid is a short small tip that shows fats, oils and sweets (ghee, butter, cream, sugar, pastries, fried and sweet preparations, like chocolates, candies, *gulab jamun, jalebi* and *ladoo*).

Alcoholic beverages are also in the same group. These foods provide extremely high calories but low vitamins and minerals. The remaining foods in all the food groups suggested in the pyramid are from low-calorie foods. The sources of proteins with high calories are not mentioned. Even carbohydrates and fruits suggested have low calories. As we are interested in weight loss, we should strictly select our food items from the substances mentioned in the pyramid to get best results.

A well-balanced diet is the way to health, fitness and wellness to live life to its fullest. About 60% of the total calories should come from carbohydrates. When you want to lose weight, you have to avoid simple carbohydrates and consume only complex carbohydrates; 20% calories from fats out of which 1/3 from saturated fats, 1/3 from polyunsaturated and 1/3 from monounsaturated fats, 20% of total calories from proteins (0.8 grams of protein per kilogram of body weight). The diet must also include all essential vitamins and minerals and 12 glasses of water.

The pyramid shows five major food groups along with fats, oils and sugars, which are used sparingly.

The pyramid suggests the following combination per day:

6–8 servings of complex carbohydrates forming the base of the pyramid (where we have tried to eliminate additional fats, sugars and processed foods)

6–8 servings of vegetables and fruits. Vegetables rich in fibers, vitamins, minerals must be selected. Fruits that are juicy, fibrous, watery, and rich in vitamin C and A are recommended.

2–3 servings of proteins. Skimmed milk, milk products, pulses, legumes, sprouts of small grams (*moong, masoor, mattki, tur*).

2–3 servings of lean meat, egg white

To achieve weight loss:

- Avoid fats, oils, sweets, sodium and alcohol.

- Increase your fiber intake.

- Eat minimum number of servings from each of the above groups.

Each meal should contain a minimum of two big bowls of vegetables and salads, 1 serving from complex carbohydrate, and 1 serving from low-cal proteins.

Word of caution: *Do not eat less than 1000 calories per day.*

Some people think that they should take vitamin supplements and mineral supplements. The population that may benefit from supplements are those with nutritional deficiencies, alcoholics, smokers, strict vegetarians, individuals with extremely low calories (less than 1000 kcal per day), older adults, new-born infants and people suffering from some diseases. External supplements are not beneficial to those who eat a healthy diet. External supplements do not help you run faster, relieve stress, jump higher, improve sexual power, boost energy levels and cure common cold.

Some special situations are discussed below. Do not consume external supplements unless recommended by your physician.

Iron: In women, iron deficiency is very common due to heavy menstrual flow, pregnancy and lactation.

Antioxidant Nutrients

Free radicals (oxidants)

Oxygen is utilized during metabolism to change carbohydrates and fats into energy. During this process, oxygen is transformed into stable forms of water and carbon dioxide. A small amount of oxygen, however, ends up in an unstable form referred to as 'oxygen-free radicals.'

A free radical has a normal proton nucleus with a single unpaired electron. Having only one electron makes the free radical extremely reactive. It is constantly looking to pair this single electron with another electron to make it paired, from any other molecule. That other molecule, which now has a single electron, becomes a free radical. This chain reaction goes on until two free radicals meet to form a stable molecule.

Free radicals attack and damage proteins and lipids, in particular cell membrane and DNA. Many times, this damage is responsible for cancer, cardiovascular disease, emphysema, cataract, Parkinson's disease and premature aging. Environmental factors such as solar radiation, cigarette smoking, air pollution, radiation, some drugs, injury or infection, chemicals and stress are responsible for formation of free radicals.

The body's own defense system neutralizes the free radicals so that they do not cause any damage. But if the rate of production of radicals is faster than that of neutralization, then they can damage the cells.

Antioxidants offer protection against free radicals in two ways.

- *They absorb free radicals before they can cause damage.*

- *They interrupt the sequence of reactions once the damage has begun.*

Taking antioxidant supplement prevents damage from free radicals. Antioxidants are found abundantly in food, especially in fruits and vegetables. Many of the benefits of antioxidants are obtained when we consume them from food sources. It is always better to have these vitamins through the diet than through supplements.

Nutrients	Source	Antioxidant effect
Vitamin C	Citrus fruits, broccoli, green, red pepper, cauliflower, cabbage, lime, guava, amla, tomatoes	Inactive free radicals
Vitamin E	Vegetable oil, green leafy vegetables, wheat germ, oat meal, almonds, cereals	Protects lipids from oxidation
Beta carotene	Carrots, pumpkin, broccoli, green leafy vegetables	Soaks oxygen-free radicals
Selenium	Seafood, meat, whole grain	Prevents damage to cell structure
Daily intake	250 to 500 mg of vitamin C 200 to 500 IU of vitamin E 10,000 to 25,000 IU of beta carotene	100 mg selenium

If you incorporate 6 servings of green salads, 2 servings of fruit with one citrus fruit, 2–3 servings of leafy vegetables daily, then you can get adequate nutrients.

But it is difficult to get vitamin E in the required amount, as it is not found in large quantities in the food consumed as part of one's diet. In such cases, supplements can be taken after advice. Vitamin E is a fat-soluble vitamin. One has to take it with some fats and in divided doses. Vitamin C is water-soluble and gets eliminated in about 12 hours. For best results, consume vitamin C rich foods twice a day or divide your vitamin C supplement into half and take them twice a day.

Vitamin E has been linked to reduced risk of heart diseases but it may not offer additional protection to people who already have the disease. Healthy people who take vitamin E have fewer heart problems. Vitamin E seems to slow down the progression of plaque in the arteries. Extra vitamin E is an anticoagulant. Therefore, the dose should be checked with the physician.

Vitamin C offers benefits against heart disease, cancer, cataract and several other health disorders. A diet rich in vitamin C is helpful. More than 500 mg is not necessary. After 200 mg, very little amounts of vitamin C is absorbed. It is better to take it twice a day (150–200 mg at a time) for maximum absorption.

Beta carotene is best obtained as a daily dose through food sources rather than through supplements. It does not offer additional health benefits to the consumer and may increase the rate of lung cancer in smokers who take beta carotene supplements. Therefore, it is recommended that you skip the pill and eat a carrot. Eating one raw carrot decreases the risk of cancers of prostate, colorectal, lung, breast, liver and digestive tract.

About 100 mg selenium per day increases energy level, decreases anxiety and improves immunity. Vitamin C and selenium should not be taken together as this hampers the absorption of vitamin C. Vitamin E should be taken with selenium as it increases the effectiveness of selenium.

Selected Food for Antioxidants

B Carotene

Rda. 10,000–25000 IU		
Apricot	One medium	675
Broccoli	1/2 cup	680
Carrot	One medium	20225
Papaya	One medium	6120
Spinach	1 and 1/2 cup	7395
Tomato	One medium	1395
Turnip	1/2 cup	3960

Vitamin C

Rda. 250–500 mg Mg		
Guava	one medium	165
Lemon juice	one lemon	110
Orange	one	120
Papaya	one	85
Pepper	1/2 cup	95
Strawberry	one cup	88
Amla	4 big	100

Vitamin E

Rda. 200 to 500 mg		IU	Mg
Almond oil	1 tsp	10.1	5.3
Peanut	25 no	3.0	
Sunflower seeds	3 tsp	14.2	
Sunflower oil	1 tsp		6.9
Wheat germ oil	1 tsp		20.0

Selenium

Rda. 100		Mcg
Whole wheat bread/*phulka*	one slice	100
Chicken breast roasted	100 g	24
Cod baked	100 g	57
Egg white boiled	one	10
Fruits	one big	1
Oatmeal	one cup	23
Salmon fish	100 g	35
Tuna	100 g	68
Walnuts	1 bowl	5
Vegetables		1

Side Effects

Vitamin E: Gastrointestinal disturbances, increase in blood lipids

Vitamin C: Nausea, diarrhea, abdominal cramps, kidney stones and liver problem

B carotene: Yellow pigmentation, contraindicated with lung cancer, smokers, alcohol

Selenium: Nausea, vomiting, diarrhea, fatigue, lesion on skin, loss of hair and nails and liver damage

In such cases, immediately stop the supplements and consult your physician.

Folate (B vitamin): Pre-menopausal and pregnant women require folate supplements. They prevent birth defects, protect colon and prevent cervical cancer.

Folate, along with BS and 812, prevents heart attacks by reducing homocysteine levels in the blood. Higher level of protein homocysteine accelerates atherosclerosis. Five servings of salads and fruit usually meet the need of nutrients. If one feels the necessity for supplements, then take the advice of your physician.

Even though you may think of taking of some supplements, fruits and vegetables are the richest sources of antioxidants and phytochemicals. Many people eating high-fat food or extra sweets feel that they should take vitamin supplements. We have to remember that supplements cannot replace any food group. Pills are no substitutes. **You have to have nutrients through your diet only.** If, in spite of a balanced diet, you suffer from any adverse health condition, only then consult your physician for supplements. Do not have them on your own. With this knowledge of basic nutrition, we have to learn the principles for weight loss and weight management.

Chapter 10

Diet Principles for Weight Reduction

Introduction

In chapter 9, we saw the basics of nutrition. Now we know the function, sources and calories provided by various food types. We are now aware of what a balanced diet is and what are the calories provided by these sources. Now let us learn to plan the diet for weight reduction. Let us see what we should consume in what proportion to fulfill our daily nutritional requirements. Which food has to be avoided? How to plan for a 1500-kcal diet, a 1200-kcal diet, and a 1000-kcal diet? What must one buy? What are the principles of adherence and so on?

Read this chapter and explore the diet menu as much as possible with various combinations. You will realize that weight-loss diet is not boring at all. On the contrary, it gives you full satisfaction along with nutrition and weight loss. So, lose your weight while enjoying food and availing yourself of nutrition.

The weaver bird weaves the nest and enjoys the job. It sings during its tedious job. Similarly, you must enjoy yourself and accept the change permanently.

We have learned that if calorie input exceeds the calorie output, the person gains weight. When calorie output is more than input, then one loses weight.

1 kg of body weight = 7600 kcal

To lose one kilogram of weight, we have to create a negative energy balance of 7600 kcal. Theoretically, it is a very simple principle but when you start your weight-loss program, you realize that the actual equation differs. If you cut 7600 kcal and achieve some weight loss without exercise, you lose your lean body mass more, rather than lose fat. The body uses protein instead of fats and carbohydrates when you cut calories without exercise. A gram of protein from the muscles has one-fifth part of protein and four-fifth of water. Loss of 1 kg protein leads to a 800-g loss of water and a 200-g loss of protein. Each kg of protein yields actually one-twentieth the amount of energy compared to a 1 kg of fat loss. As a result, most of the weight loss is water loss, which on the scale looks very good.

Exercise, along with a low-calorie balanced diet, is the best method for weight loss. We have already discussed that exercise plays an important role in weight loss. Along with exercise, the role of diet is equally important to achieve and maintain the lost weight. We learned the set point theory, the plateau theory and weight cycling in detail. Along with a scientific exercise regimen, a scientific way of diet plan is necessary. The daily calorie intake should not be less than 1200 calories. **Weight is gained over many years. So, for weight loss, adequate time should be given.**

A diet cannot be viewed as a temporary tool to aid weight loss but it should be considered as a permanent change in eating behavior, to ensure weight management and better health. While chalking out your diet plan, you have to find out the calorie input by taking into consideration all the small details of your food intake—from the first cup of tea in the morning till the last serving of food before going to bed. You have to take into consideration the caloric expenditure every day. For this, you have to calculate your basal metabolism rate first. We know that basal metabolism rate is the amount of energy (calories) required by the body, while at rest, to perform the vital functions of heart beat, respiration, maintenance of body temperature and cellular function.

Given below is a simple formula to calculate BMR.

Rough calculation for BMR

Harris-Benedict's Equation

Males: $66 + (13.7 \times W) + (5 \times H) - (6.8 \times A)$.
Females: $65.5 + (9.6 \times W) + (1.7 \times H) - (4.7 \times A)$.

W – Weight in kilograms
H – Height in centimeters
A – Age in years

The calculations are approximations. BMR accounts for two-thirds of the body's daily need for calories. The remaining one-third amount is required for all other activities just to maintain the person at the current weight he or she is having. Now you are aware of your BMR. The next step is to get the knowledge of the additional calorie expenditure by the exercise that you do. You have calculated the calories you are expending every day. Now, you have to calculate the quantum of calories you need to consume to create a negative energy balance.

For planning your diet, you have to cut the unwanted calories from junk food. Simultaneously, you have to take care that you are including all the nutrients in the recommended dietary allowance and the total count is not less than 1200 kcal per day. If you are consuming 2800 kcal per day, you have to cut the additional fats, sugar and alcohol, which are simple empty calories that get immediately absorbed and stored without expending much calories on them. This means the thermic effect of such food is very low. You can eliminate around 400 kcal per day through such a deduction.

Through increased calorie output by exercise, scientifically designed as per the guidelines discussed in last chapter, you can utilize an additional 400 kcal per day.

Now, the total negative calorie balance will be around 800 kcal per day. In ten days, 8000 kcal negative energy balance will be achieved. This will lead to a weight reduction of about 1 kg in 10 days and 3 kg in 30 days. To help you monitor and adhere to your diet plan, you have to maintain the record of daily food intake. These guidelines are developed from the food guide pyramid and the recommended dietary allowance guidelines discussed earlier. The objective is to match the number of servings allowed in each plan.

Every time you eat as per the chart, you have to just record it in your diary for that day. Now you have to select the plan, after taking into consideration your BMR, calorie input and calorie output through physical activity and exercise.

- Calculate 25 calories from 1 bowl vegetables (raw)

Salient Features of the Daily Diet Plan for Weight Reduction

- Have four meals a day.

- Breakfast before 9 a.m. is the first meal. For breakfast, have two servings of food containing the following

    1. Complex carbohydrate: cereals, any type of bread (phulka/khakara/idli/plain dosa/small uttappam/paratha/thepla/brown bread), porridge of daliya/ragi flour/oats/millets/quinoa, 100 grams of cooked unpolished rice or 100 grams of cooked wheat pasta

    2. One serving of protein: One cup of milk/curds/buttermilk/thin dal/100 gm. i.e. ½ bowl of sprouts/100 gm. tofu/2 egg whites/100 gm lean meat

    3. Two big bowls of salads

- Lunch before 1 p.m. is the second meal. It must have two servings of complex carbohydrates, two servings of proteins and two big bowls of salads.

- Third meal at 4 p.m.: 1) one fruit 2) 4 almonds, 4 walnuts 3) a cheese cube and 4) green tea

- Fourth meal at 7 p.m.: 1) one serving of carbohydrates 2) one serving of protein 3) two bowls of salads

When you start a particular plan, you have to be careful about the size of bowl or cup.

1 cup serving = 200 ml

1 glass = 300 ml

1 bowl = 200ml

- Read the labels carefully.

Calories from dietary fats, sugar, alcohol or junk food are more easily converted to body fat. Fat requires less energy to be converted to triglycerides. If you consume calories from such foods, then it becomes very difficult to lose weight. There are so many preparations that contain hidden fats. You have to avoid food substances like ghee, butter, sweet and fried preparations, pizza, burger, *paneer,* cheese, nuts, refined products, instant noodles, dry fruits, chocolates, milkshakes, ice cream, puddings, pastries, fruit juices, sugarcane juice, soft drinks, cold drinks, hard drinks, *sago,* potato chips, fried peanuts, red meat, Punjabi dishes with rich gravies, and Chinese dishes with oil, which have lots of hidden calories.

Fruits that have to be restricted are mango, sapota, banana, grapes, pineapple, custard apple and jackfruit, basically those with less fiber and more pulp and those that are very sweet.

Vegetables having less fibers, *yam, taro root,* brinjal and potato must be restricted. Have ample vegetables, as much as possible, from the remaining vegetables in the group.

Fruits that contain more fiber and are juicy and watery are to be taken in large quantities. Pulses, legumes, sprouts like *chhole, rajma, harbhare, chawali,* peas and beans are to be restricted, while *moong, masoor, matki* and *toor* are to be taken in large quantities. When sprouts are developed longer, protein content increases.

Things You Must Remember

- Eat lots of salads and vegetables (at least two big bowls) before every meal.

- Drink lots of water, preferably 10–12 glasses through the day.

- Drink buttermilk, tender coconut water, vegetable juices, soups and other healthy drinks through the day.

- Avoid tea and coffee and in-between snacking.

- Use minimum amount of oil or ghee in cooking.

- Avoid cooking with coconut, peanut, sesame and poppy seeds.

- Avoid sugar, jaggery and honey. You can use stevia leaves.

- Use skimmed milk, 1/2 a liter every day, pulses, egg white, or lean meat.

- Avoid fried preparations or preparations with lot of oil and ghee.

- Have a variety of the allowed foods and enjoy the meal by adding spices and trying out different combinations.

- Chew the food very well till it gets converted into liquid paste.

- Have the food at the same place every day.

- Use a smaller dish.

- Have small and frequent meals.

- Breakfast should be the first meal of the day. Do not skip breakfast. Breakfast is an awakening call to the metabolism. Remember this old wise saying. *Breakfast like a king, lunch like a citizen and supper like a pauper.* Consume 70% of the total daily calorie requirement by 2–3 p.m. Only 30% of calories should be consumed at dinner.

- Dinner should be light and early, preferably around 7 p.m.

- If you feel hungry after dinner, you can have clear vegetable soups and salads.

- While eating out, opt for lunch than a late dinner. Consume lots of salad before setting out for dinner. Order for clear veg soup, *tandoori roti* and preparations with less oil.

When you are on a weight-loss program, after any lapse in the diet plan, you immediately put on the lost weight. It takes eight days to come back to the original lost weight you had before the lapse. It's better to avoid eating out at restaurants and parties. Learn to deny humbly. Do not say yes, when you want to say no. At restaurants, the words 'baked,' 'grilled,' 'boiled,' 'tandoor,' 'smoked,' 'steamed,' 'poached' and 'flame cooked' are used. But additional fats are used for palatability. You have to take care and instruct the people at the hotel to not any additional oil.

Appetizers and soups: Choose clear vegetarian soup without any butter, oil, ghee, corn flour or sugar at a restaurant. A fruit plate with juicy watery fruits, without sugar and salts, must be eaten. Boiled, steamed, tandoori starters, without hidden fats, can be ordered.

Entrees: Select seafood and chicken dishes made using low-calorie methods, without coconut, peanut, butter, cashew paste and dry fruits.

Ask for the ingredients. Suggest your recipe or modifications in the restaurant's recipe and get what suits you. For example, ask for mixed vegetables without cashew powder, cream and butter and with very less oil and spices. Avoid sour cream and butter.

Salads use vinegar or lime juice and spices as dressing. Ask for the dressing to be served separately.

Sandwiches: Choose low-calorie fillings with lots of salads, without cheese and butter.

Beverages: Choose iced water, tea or coffee without sugar or cream, instead of alcoholic beverages. Choose lentils, kabab and tandoor vegetables, instead of deep-fried snacks.

Daily Diet Menus

Model diet plan supplying 1000 kcal per day

Early morning 1 glass of lukewarm water + juice of half a lemon

Morning breakfast 7 a.m. to 9.30 a.m.

- 2 big bowls of salad/vegetables, raw/cooked/stir fried with or without spices; or 1 glass of vegetable juice/smoothie

- Any two servings of complex carbohydrate group namely any type of bread or ½ bowl of porridge of ragi/oats/½ bowl of preparations of quinoa, oats or any grain/cereal

- Any one serving from this protein group. 1 cup of skimmed milk/1 cup of curds/1 glass of buttermilk, ½ cup of sprouts/½ cup of soy chunk granules/100 g of tofu/2 egg whites/100 g of chicken or fish (boiled, tandoor, steamed or grilled)

Lunch 11.30 a.m. to 2.30 p.m.

2 big bowls of salad + 2 servings out of complex carbohydrate group + 2 servings out of protein group

Late afternoon 3 p.m. to 6 p.m.

1 fruit + tender coconut water

Dinner around 7 p.m.

2 big bowls of salad + 1 serving of protein + 1 serving of complex carbohydrate + 1 big bowl of clear vegetable soup

9 p.m. – 1 big bowl of clear vegetable soup

Tips for Behavioral Modification and Adherence to a Lifetime Weight Management Program

Achieving and maintaining the recommended body composition is by no means impossible but it requires desire and commitment. To make your dream true, you have to retain the changed lifestyle. It is crucial for success. Modifying old habits and developing new, positive and permanent changes take time. To commit yourself to a healthy lifestyle forever, you can try these tips.

- **Make a commitment to change:** The desire to modify your lifestyle is the first step. Do not remain in a 'to be or not to be' phase. You have to realize that, for the sake of good health and quality of life, you have to change and to be successful, your sincere commitment is extremely necessary. The desire to lose weight must be stronger than the desire to overeat and miss the exercise session.

- **Set realistic goals:** As we have already discussed, goals must be realistic. Realize that, over the period of years, you have become overweight and it is going to take a longer period to lose the substantial amount of weight. The long-term goal of 25 kg in a year is realistic. This should be accompanied by shorter goals of loss of one kg per 10 days for the first two months.

- **Incorporate exercise** into the program as discussed earlier. A scientific exercise regime under supervision is an important aspect of weight loss and weight management.

- **Differentiate hunger and appetite:** Hunger is the actual physical need of food. Appetite is the desire of food usually triggered by factors such as stress, habits, boredom, depression, availability of food and just the thought of food itself. You decide to eat only when you have a physical need. You have to develop and stick to a regular meal pattern.

- **Eat less fat**, as each gram of fat provides 9 kcal. Each gram of protein and carbohydrates provide only 4 kcal. Cutting fats means cutting more calories with each meal.

- **When you cut fat** and start consuming low-fat food, **you have to restrict the total food intake as well.** You must not be under the impression that you can eat a low-fat diet in whatever quantity you want

- **Cut out unnecessary items from your diet:** Many people are habitual of eating fried chips, salted cashew or peanuts while reading or watching TV. Some people feel that drinking *sherbet* in afternoon is a very healthy habit. Some people like to eat chocolate/sweets after a meal. Drinking an energy drink after exercise, as shown in TV advertisements, tends to impress so many people. But this is not right. Pastries, wafers, *samosas*, cakes, and chips are carried by children in their lunch box along with the recommended nutritious snacks. This must be avoided. Avoiding 200 extra calories per day amounts to avoiding 10 kg fats per year.

- **Learn to overcome physiological craving:** Many people have a biological imbalance of insulin. Insulin helps the body 'use and conserve energy.' Some people produce so much insulin that their body cannot use it at all. This imbalance leads to an overpowering craving for carbohydrates. Consuming more carbohydrates leads to release of more insulin from the body. To reduce craving, we have to have proteins and non-starchy vegetables. Foods like egg white, fish, chicken, tofu, lettuce, broccoli, mushroom and sprouts reduce craving.

- **Avoid automatic eating:** Consuming 1–2 spoons of sugar while preparing tea, eating peanuts and coconut while grinding them, licking butter while preparing buttermilk, eating chips while watching TV, eating popcorn while watching movies in the theater, and eating ice cream passing through the play park are all common habits. Most of the time, food consumed during such events lack nutritional value and are high in calories.

- **Stay busy** during a weight-reduction program. Even otherwise, keep yourself busy. When you sit around and do nothing, you tend to eat more. Occupying the mind and body with activities, not related to eating, helps take away the desire to eat. Try something new and exciting. Some options are playing sports, sewing, knitting, visiting the museum, exhibitions, park and library, walking, cycling, playing, gardening, going to hobby classes or a beauty salon, painting, and doing social work. They help break the monotony of life and you may develop useful skills.

- **Plan meals ahead of time**: Sensible shopping is necessary to accomplish this objective. Always shop after meals. This will help you stay away from unhealthy foods and snack on the way home. The shopping list should include only the things that you can eat, so that you do not get tempted and impulsive to buy unwanted stuff.

- **Cook wisely**

  ➢ Use less fat and refined/instant products.

  ➢ Trim all the visible fats from meat.

  ➢ Remove skin from poultry.

  ➢ Skim the fat off gravies and soups.

  ➢ Bake, boil, broil, steam, grill and tandoor instead of frying and shallow frying.

  ➢ Avoid butter, cream, mayonnaise and salad dressing oils to garnish the preparations.

  ➢ Use non-stick frying pans.

  ➢ Prepare recipes that contain plenty of fibers.

  ➢ Do not sieve whole wheat flour.

  ➢ Use a variety of vegetables from all seasons in various colors.

  ➢ Use iron utensils to cook vegetables.

  ➢ Try to get maximum sprouts for legumes.

  ➢ Eat fruits as desserts.

  ➢ Stay away from soda pop, fruit juices, fruit flavored drinks and cold drinks.

  ➢ Do not use any syrups or *sherbets*.

  ➢ Drink plenty of water throughout the day.

➤ Eat lots of salads and soups prior to a meal.

➤ Eat early and have a light dinner.

- **Do not serve yourself more food than you should eat**. Measure the food in portions and keep serving bowls away from table. This way, you will eat less, have a harder time getting second helpings and have a lesser appetite because food is not visible. Do not force anybody, especially children when they say they have had enough.

- **Try junior size** instead of senior size. Use smaller plates, bowls, cups and glasses. Eat half as much food as you typically eat. Over the year, the sizes of dishes and glasses have got bigger. Consequently, one eats a lot more than one needs. If you use a smaller plate, it will look like you are having more food and you will tend to eat less. Even in restaurants, more food is served. Even after eating is over, people carry home leftovers. The size of cold drink bottles is also increasing day by day.

- **Eat out infrequently:** The more you eat out, the more you consume extra calories. Every time you consume 300 kcal extra, 30% more fats is being added to your body.

- **Eat slowly and eat sitting at the table only.** Eating is one of the pleasures of life and we need to take time to enjoy it. Eating on the run is not good. The body does not get time to register the nutritive and calorie consumption. You overeat before the body perceives the fullness. Eating at the table also demands some time to eat; it deters snacking between meals. This is because, every time you want to eat, you have to come to the table, sit down and eat. When the eating is done, do not continue sitting at the table. Get up, clean up and put away the food to stop further eating.

- **Avoid social binges.** Social gatherings are difficult events to stop yourself from eating, especially when you see everybody around you eating. Plan ahead and visualize yourself in the place. Do not get pressured to eat or drink. Do not rationalize in these situations. Choose low-cal food and entertain yourself with other activities such as dancing and talking. Do not forget to eat lots of salads at home before going to the party. At the party, have salad and soup, followed by low-cal foods. Remember, the party is for sharing joy not only for eating and drinking.

- **Do not store the edible stuff with high calories** in the refrigerator or on the grocery shelves in the kitchen. Do not bring home high-calorie, high-sugar or high-fat food. If they are there for others, store them where they are hard to see or reach. If they are out of sight or not readily available, the temptation to eat is less. Keep the food on the highest shelf or in the storeroom, under a lock and key, as this needs additional efforts to access. Do not entirely avoid the treats, but consume them in limited quantities.

- **Avoid evening food raids:** Most people with weight problems do really well during the day but lose it at night time. Excessive snacking followed by an evening meal is a common pitfall. Stay busy after supper. Go for a short walk and go to bed early. Good rest at night helps conquer the intense desire for food during the evening hours.

- **Make eating pleasurable** by eating slowly, focusing on pleasing and relaxing conversations, mild humor. Create a caring atmosphere.

- **Practice stress management techniques** (next chapter). If you are used to eating as a solution to fight stress, then the first thing you have to do is to learn ways to manage stress. Eating is not a stress-releasing activity. It aggravates the problem if weight control is the issue.

- **Get support:** Find friends, colleagues and family members who support your weight-loss program. Form a support group of people like you. The more support you receive, the better you will perform.

- **Monitor changes and reward accomplishments.** Losing weight is a reward in itself. The changes in your lifestyle deserve recognition. You have started liking the exercise, you have changed your diet, you are regular in your treatment, you are changing your lifestyle, you are achieving some success every day and there is countable weight loss every month. These are situations that must be rewarded definitely. A new pair of shoes, new clothing, a new track suit or a new piece of jewelry can be the rewards for your success, which was achieved through determination even though it was difficult.

- **Prepare for lapses:** Do not splurge even though you slip up. Do not despair and give up. Reevaluate and continue your efforts. You may commit mistakes being a trying personality. Only those who try can make mistakes. Learn from the mistakes and improve. An occasional slip will not punish you by gaining what you have lost. At such a time, do not get tempted to do the same thing again and again. Making mistake is human and it does not mean failure.

- **Positive mental attitude** is the key to success. Avoid negative thoughts, negative past experiences, negative environment and negative people around you. Instead, think of all benefits you will reap, such as feeling, looking and functioning better, enjoying better health and improving your quality of life. Relapses are inevitable. Failure comes to those who give up; do not use previous experiences to build upon and develop skills that will prevent self-defeating behavior in future.

Where there is a will, there is way. Those who persist will reap the reward.

Food You Must Incorporate in Your Diet as Protective Food

Fruits

Apples contain soluble fibers. They boost the production of enzymes that make carcinogens (cancer causing) more soluble in water and aid in eliminating them from body. They bind nitrates in the stomach.

Nitrates cannot get converted into nitrosamines, which are carcinogenic. Apples have a protective factor that can protect us from Parkinson's disease.

Apricots contain six carotenoids, which help prevent various forms of cancers.

Citrus fruits like orange, sweet lime, lemon and grape fruit contain anti-cancer carotenoid that helps prevent lung cancer and help in the elimination of carcinogens.

Fig contains an anti-cancer substance. It also helps prevent psoriasis.

Papaya is an antioxidant that contains beta carotene. It provides anti-cancerous benefits.

Strawberries contain a cholesterol-reducing substance.

Watermelon contains an anti-cancer substance.

- **Fresh vegetables**

  Broccoli has an anti-cancer substance that prevent damage of cell DNA.

  Cabbage prevents development of lung cancer.

  Carrots have an antioxidant.

  Celery prevents psoriasis and lymphoma.

  Pumpkin has an anti-cancer property.

  Spinach has an anti-cancer property.

  Tomatoes are anti-cancer and anti-hypertensive.

- **Whole grains**

  Oats, whole wheat, and millet provide healthy and protective soluble and insoluble fibers, anti-cancer mineral selenium, anti-cancer and heart risk-reducing factors.

  Oats contain GABA, which is a tonic to the brain.

- **Legumes**

  Legumes are beneficial to diabetics for balancing insulin, stabilizing blood sugar, metabolizing excess fats and keeping LDL low. They have anti-cancer properties.

- **Omega 3 fatty acid sources**

  Fishes salmon, tuna, mackerel, green leafy vegetables, broccoli, soy, tofu and walnut.

- **Yogurt** is anti-cancerous.

- **Selected spices and herbs**

  Garlic and onions prevent cancer and heart disease.

  Black pepper and mustard improve metabolic rate, increase fat-burning capacity, has anti-cancerous, anti-migraine properties, and protect against arthritis, asthma and bronchitis.

  Cinnamon and **turmeric** triple the ability of insulin to metabolize glucose.

  Basil, cumin and turmeric boost immunity, prevent cancers and boost the ability to utilize insulin.

- Buy fresh and clean food.

- Cover pans when boiling or steaming to preserve nutrients and energy.

- Wash fresh vegetables and fruits before eating, to remove dirt, harmful bacteria and chemical residues.

- Avoid moldy foods.

- Avoid foods that have a stale smell, discoloration or an old appearance.

- Fish and flesh should be cleaned properly. Cut them on a wooden board instead of plastic to avoid bacteria. Cook them thoroughly to kill bacteria.

- Say no to burned and barbequed foods. If you have to consume them, avoid high-fat mixes, charred material and smoked contact. (Wrap it in foil while cooking.)

Some Special Conditions in Women

Osteoporosis

Osteo means 'bone porosis,' which means brittleness. Brittleness of the bones due to loss in bone mass is called osteoporosis. This increases the risk of bone fracture. Primarily, the bones of hip, wrist and spine become weak and brittle and get fractured easily. The process begins slowly in the third or fourth decade of life. Women are especially susceptible after menopause, because of loss of estrogen. Estrogen helps absorb calcium; deficiency of estrogen leads to increased rate of osteoporosis. That is why women are eight times more susceptible to this condition than men.

Osteoporosis is diagnosed only after the occurrence of fracture. Day by day, the percentage of women suffering from this condition is increasing. Fracture of the hip bone is very common and 50% of elderly women do not recover from it. They either become dependent on others in later life or they die within six months.

Osteoporosis Is Preventable

The risk factors of this disease are inadequate calcium intake, sedentary lifestyle, excessive intake of alcohol, caffeine and phosphorus through soft drinks, and cigarette smoking. Other reasons are low estrogen level at the age of menopause. Extremely thin women are also susceptible to osteoporosis.

Sources of Calcium

	Measure	Weight in mg
Skimmed milk	1 cup	216
Low-fat cheese	½ cup	78
Oat meal	½ cup	109
Yogurt	1 cup	448
Soy milk	1 cup	400
Tofu	½ cup	138
Cabbage	1 cup	158
Broccoli	1 cup	72
Orange	1 cup	75
Spinach	1 cup	56
Turnip	1 cup	197
Drumstick	100 gm	200
Amaranth	100 gm	200
Finger Millet	100 gm	200

Adequate calcium intake and exercise are simple ways to prevent osteoporosis. The recommended daily calcium intake is 1000 mg for adults and 1500 mg for post-menopausal women. If you take sufficient dairy products with raw vegetables and fruits, diet alone can fulfill the calcium requirements. If required, calcium supplements can be taken after medical advice. They should be taken on an empty stomach, a minimum of 30 minutes before any food. It is always advisable to consume calcium-rich food than consume calcium supplements.

Exercise improves bone density. It plays a key role in prevention of osteoporosis. It prevents bone loss following menopause. Gym exercises are extremely useful in prevention of osteoporosis. The origin and insertion of muscle is in the bone; whatever impact you take on the muscle through resistance, it gets transferred to the bone as well. Bones get stronger; even ligaments, tendons and muscles become stronger. This improves the stability of joints and the support of skeleton. Exercises also improve balance and coordination, which can help prevent falls and injuries. Active people have denser bone minerals. To have good bone health, it is necessary to participate in regular physical activity.

Estrogen is the most important factor in preventing bone loss, especially at the lumbar region. After menopause, a good diet rich in calcium and regular gym exercises is the best combination. It has been proven to help prevent bone loss. If you have been doing gym exercises from the age of 30, it is more beneficial. Estrogen replacement therapy (ERT) promotes bone density if taken over a long term. ERT also reduces the risk of cardiovascular disease. However, ERT has unpleasant side effects that include headaches, breast tenderness, bleeding and fluid retention. ERT may lead to breast cancer too.

New treatment modalities to prevent bone loss, like selective estrogen receptor modalities (SERM), is an upcoming boon. Unlike ERT, these compounds have a positive effect on blood lipids, prevent bone loss and pose no risk to breast and uterine tissue.

Iron Deficiency (Anemia)

Iron is a vital nutrient for many cell activities and a key element of hemoglobin in the blood. Hemoglobin carries oxygen to tissues from the lungs via blood. Iron is also a constituent of myoglobin, which holds a small amount of oxygen in muscle tissues.

The RDA (recommended dietary allowance) for women is 18 mg per day. People who do not have sufficient iron in their diet can develop iron deficiency anemia. Because of less iron, hemoglobin reduces and then sufficient oxygen is not carried to the blood tissue. This leads to reduced endurance, early and frequent fatigue, and increased susceptibility to cold and infections.

Inadequate iron intake, blood loss through menstruation, physical activity, heavy training, and extensive jogging lead to iron deficiency. The rates of iron absorption and iron loss vary from person to person. Iron sources in food occur in two forms: heam iron and non-heam iron. Heam iron is found only in foods derived from animal flesh. Non-heam iron is found in both plant and animal foods. The rate of heam iron absorption is better than that of non-heam. People can get enough iron by eating iron-rich foods such as green leafy vegetables, enriched grain products, egg, fish and lean meat. Organ meat and red meat are also good sources, but they are high in cholesterol and it is better to avoid them.

Name	Quantity	Iron (mg)
Broccoli	½ cup	1.4
Spinach raw	1 cup	1.7
Fenugreek	1 cup	1.7
Vegetables mixed	1 cup	2.4
Finger Millet	100 gm	7.2
Apple	1	1.8
Fig	1	1.1
Sprouts with skin	1 cup	4.4

- Use iron utensils.

- Boil curry in an iron pan.

- Use an iron knife to cut vegetables.

This amount of knowledge about nutrition and diet will help you reduce the risk of developing certain chronic diseases. We can summarize the guidelines for your health and that of your family thus:

A – Aim for fitness.

- Aim for healthy weight.

- Avoid habits of alcohol and smoking.

B – Be physically active every day.

- Build a healthy base.

C – Choose foods based on the pyramid guide.

- Choose a variety of whole grains.

- Choose a variety of fruits and vegetables daily.

- Choose foods that are safe to eat.

- Choose sensibly.

- Choose a diet low in saturated fat and cholesterol and moderate in total fat.

- Choose beverages and foods that minimize your intake of sugars.

- Choose and prepare foods with moderate salt.

Achieving weight loss is not as difficult as retaining it and following a nutrition plan for life.

No single food can provide all the necessary nutrients and other beneficial substances in the amount that the body needs. You have to combine a variety of nutrients and other substances needed for good health.

An ounce of prevention is worth a pound of cure. The sooner you implement the dietary guidelines presented here, the better are your chances of preventing chronic diseases and reaching higher state of wellness. You have to keep repeating and reminding yourself that the commitment to a healthy lifestyle is a commitment for your entire lifetime.

Alcohol

Alcohol consumption is closely related to obesity. 1 gm of alcohol provides 7 kcal, which is double when compared to carbohydrates. The TEF of alcohol is negligible. It immediately gets absorbed in the blood and gets stored as additional calories. The snacks and dinner generally consumed with alcohol are fried and calorie rich.

People drink alcohol for many reasons. In small amounts and for short periods of time, alcohol relieves tension, encourages a sense of wellbeing and is unlikely to be harmful. However, some people mistakenly use alcohol to relieve major problems. There are subtle social pressures to drink. Slowly, the alcohol consumed loosens the tongue and convinces people that their social interactions can be improved. Presentation of alcoholic beverages can reinforce this pressure by implying that the product will make you not only socially acceptable but also attractive interesting and desirable. There may even be a suggestion that alcohol enables you to do things you could not do before. People also reward themselves by drinking. They drink to fill in empty hours, relieve tiredness, lethargy, anxiety or stress. Some people find that an alcoholic drink is the ultimate solution to all their problems.

In the liver, alcohol gets oxidized. A small portion gets exhaled and/or excreted via the urine. Alcohol is a demon drink. During weight loss, it causes many slips especially during weekends, which wipes out all the efforts done throughout the week.

Alcohol is probably the most difficult habit to curb. It is relatively high in calories and makes big inroads into your daily calorie amounts. It does not contain any nutrients, so it has no food value. Consequently, you get fat and malnourished. Alcohol must be referred to by its real name—intoxicating liquor. The word 'toxic' should remind you of its poisonous effects on the body—aggression and violence in the short term and liver damage, ulcers, high blood pressure, depression, sexual difficulties and brain damage in the long term.

Apart from the high-calorie content, it can have another drawback during weight loss and maintenance. Firstly, alcohol takes effect in your body quickly because of your low-cal intake throughout the day. Secondly, it impairs judgment. So, you tend to overeat while under its influence. Thirdly, the subsequent hangover may lead you to consoling yourself with unnecessary food.

It is better to completely avoid alcohol in your diet. Say no firmly. *Do not say yes when you want to say no.*

The following chart will help you to measure the calories through alcoholic drinks.

Sherry sweet	30 ml	43 kcal
Brandy 40% proof	30 ml	65 kcal
Gin 40% proof	30 ml	65 kcal
Rum 40% proof	30 ml	65 kcal
Vodka 40% proof	30 ml	65 kcal
Whiskey 40% proof	30 ml	65 kcal
Red wine	100 ml	68 kcal
White wine sweet	100 ml	94 kcal
Beer	100 ml	40 kcal

Note: 30 ml is a small peg.

In a healthy lifestyle, alcohol does not have any space at all.

Smoking

The younger generation is under the false notion that smoking helps lose weight by reducing appetite. They also believe that smoking helps lose the fat on the cheeks. Well, smoking will never help you lose weight. As we have learned earlier, exercise and a balanced nutritious diet are the basic factors for weight loss. With smoking, weight reduction will never happen. On the contrary, you will commit to life-threatening disorders like cancer and heart disease. Almost every system of the body gets adversely affected by smoking.

Once you get trapped into nicotine, then it is extremely difficult to escape from it. The goal of weight loss for health will remain a dream and you will be faced with life-threatening consequences. Avoid risky behavior that destroys the quality of life. You have to learn the facts about habits, so that you can make a choice with responsibility. You have to protect yourself as well as your near and dear ones from the startling effects of secondary smoking. Say no to alcohol, retrain yourself from smoking or any substance abuse and prevent yourself from any bad habit. These are the key words for averting both physical as well as psychological damage.

Chapter 11

Rest and Relaxation

Introduction

Thorough information about sleep and techniques to get a sound sleep, to give rest to your brain and to improve its efficiency are given in this chapter. Simultaneously, this chapter also discusses in detail stress, the most dangerous risk factor of health. Simple techniques that will help you analyze your vulnerability to stress and its management techniques are discussed briefly. Have good rest and proper relaxation and keep away stress and stress-related disorders. Remember, you can lose weight more easily when you are happy. Be happy and lose weight; lose weight and be happy!

The third and important aspect of a healthy lifestyle is rest and relaxation. Everybody likes to rest. Sleep is the best mode of relaxation. Sleep is extremely necessary to give proper rest to our body and mind. Sleep is an essential activity for fitness and wellbeing and vice versa. A healthy lifestyle is an essential aspect of sleep. Even the feeling of being deprived of sleep can cause symptoms similar to lack of sleep.

We all covet a good sleep. It is a natural, deep and refreshing experience and a way to revitalize our personal power. Sleep is interwoven with every facet of our daily life. It affects our health and wellbeing, our moods and behavior, our energy and emotions, our married lives and jobs, and our very sanity and happiness.

Sleep protects the brain. A deep rejuvenating sleep promotes peak brain function because, at that time, the brain gets good rest.

During sleep, your brain reinforces memories and makes sense of your daily experience, through an extra-neural activity. During sleep, proteins are manufactured by nerve cells. These proteins are similar to proteins that are produced by the stimulation from brain exercise. Such proteins help restore cellular memories. Thus, sleep is necessary to retain cellular memory and sort out the information input from the preceding hours. The amount of sleep varies from person to person. It is normally between 5 to 8 hours. Actually, quality of sleep is more important than quantity. Going into deep sleep as soon as you wish to is an indicator of good health. Physically active people, who do good exercise and consume good food, get sleep immediately. Whereas lack of physical activity, intake of unwanted food in unwanted quantity, tension, worries and stress lead to disturbance of sleep.

Sleep is a good tool to become stress-free. During sleep, the blood supply is diverted toward the digestive system. Digestion takes place and nutrients are supplied for metabolism. The body's repair work is taken care of during sleep. The brain gets rest from continuous work of coping with situations like collecting knowledge, analyzing it, taking decisions, giving orders, thinking, rethinking, changing plans, creating new things, enjoying good things, and trying to cope up with unpleasant situations. Rest to the brain is extremely essential. The brain, after good rest, works with full efficiency, with new creations and thoughts to deal with situations. Depending upon your sleep pattern, your basic level of anxiety varies. If you do not have a sleep problem, you can remain calm in most situations with a low arousal. If you lie awake with an alert and anxious mind at night, then you will become a worrier and get highly aroused. An empty mind is a devil's workshop. If the worry is short-term, then it may cause temporary insomnia (sleeplessness). The normal sleep pattern is resumed as soon as the problem is solved. Sometimes, anxiety can lead to more sleep to escape from the problem.

There are certain dos and don'ts that may help people get sleep.

- **Exercise regularly:** Physical exertion due to exercise leads to good sleep. Due to exercise, happy hormones, like endorphins, get secreted from the brain, which leads to a calming effect and a good sleep. Exercise is the best mode of relaxation (we will discuss this in stress management). Exercise increases the strength of the mind along with the strength of the body. This helps overcome anxiety.

- **Get up early:** Set the body clock as per nature. Get up at sunrise and keep on working throughout the day, return home by evening, have a good relaxed hour after an early dinner, and go to bed earlier than usual. Remember, early to bed and early to rise makes a person healthy, fit and wise.

- **Be regular** every day. Try to follow the same good habits each night. It is important to get up early every day.

- **Be happy** before sleep. Revise the good things and achievements you had throughout the day, in the last week, in the last month, in the last year, in the last few years, in your life till tonight.

- **Be thankful** to everybody who has helped you in your achievements and to God. **Pray** before going to sleep.

- **Set and follow a pre-sleep routine** like light exercise followed by a hot bath, a warm drink and a short period of reading.

- **Learn meditation.** About 15 minutes of meditation is as beneficial as eight hours of sleep.

- **Think positive,** be positive and get positive health.

Now let us learn to relax by managing our stress.

Stress Management

We are living in a modern world of fast progress. Busy schedules, peer pressure at the workplace, new challenges, and competitions are some of the classic features of the world today. These features are required to succeed in this modern world. To some extent, these requirements are useful but when you get carried away unknowingly by the unavoidable, unmanageable and overambitious demands of your big dreams, you unwillingly allow the problem of stress to enter your life. Stress is a fact of modern life. Stress masks your physical and psychological behavior and works adversely on your health. Over time, stress becomes **distress** and brings down your efficiency, productivity and health.

Obesity is one of the chronic distresses caused by stress. The weight-reduction program becomes a stressful event if it is not performed in a scientific way, as described in this book. This shows that stress leads to obesity and obesity leads to stress. Like obesity, stress also leads to various chronic health disorders like CAD, diabetes, hypertension, eating disorders, ulcers, asthma, depression, migraine, headaches, chronic fatigues and development of certain types of cancers.

The most important aspect of the treatment of obesity is managing the stress. This will help you lose weight and maintain it and protect you from stress-related disorders. It is crucial to recognize when stress becomes distress and overcome the problem, quickly and effectively.

The encouraging fact is stress can be self-controlled. You have to accept that stress is a normal part of life and you have to deal with it and learn to cope up effectively. You should not try to avoid it entirely, as a certain amount of stress is necessary for optimum health, performance and wellbeing. It is difficult to succeed and have fun in life without' hits, runs and errors.' Somebody has very rightly said that stress is like salt in food, without which food cannot be enjoyed and excess of which spoils the food.

Stress is the body's mental, emotional and physiological response to any situation that is exciting, new, threatening or frightening.

The body responds to stress in a rapid-fire sequence of physical changes known as 'fight or flight.'

When stress is positive i.e. **eustress**, the body performs in a better way and there is improvement in the health. When stress is negative i.e. distress, both health and performance begin to deteriorate. Generally, a person with type A personality has more chances of getting stressed. The peculiarities of type A personality people are:

- Uncontrollable urge to compete

- Tendency to get angry, irritated or aggravated

- Tendency to interrupt others when they are communicating

- Speak loudly and forcefully

- Show impatience and aggression

- Cannot tolerate delay, indiscipline and imperfection

You have to analyze yourself and find out whether you belong to type A personality group or not. It is observed that type A people become obese easily. While managing weight, we have to learn to manage stress. We know that, like obesity, stress too has the potential to cause various life-threatening disorders. Just like stress leads to obesity, obesity also leads to stress. By managing stress, we can manage obesity; likewise, management of obesity manages stress.

Let us first find out your vulnerability to stress with the help of the following questionnaire.

	Strongly agree	Mildly agree	Mildly disagree	Strongly Disagree
1. I try to incorporate as much as physical activity in my routine as possible.	1	2	3	4
2. I exercise aerobically for 20 minutes, at least 3 times a week.	1	2	3	4
3. I regularly sleep for 7 to 8 hours every night.	1	2	3	4
4. I have at least 1 hot, balanced meal a day.	1	2	3	4
5. I consume fewer than 2 cups of tea or coffee a day.	1	2	3	4
6. I have a recommended body weight.	1	2	3	4
7. I enjoy good health.	1	2	3	4
8. I do not use tobacco in any form.	1	2	3	4
9. I limit my alcohol intake or try to avoid it totally.	1	2	3	4
10. I do not use hard drugs (chemical dependency).	1	2	3	4
11. I have someone I love and I trust their help in taking decision.	1	2	3	4
12. There is love in my family.	1	2	3	4
13. I routinely give and receive affection.	1	2	3	4
14. I respect the person giving me security.	1	2	3	4
15. I have guides to give me good advice.	1	2	3	4
16. I can openly discuss problems with people whom I trust.	1	2	3	4
17. Other people rely on me for help.	1	2	3	4
18. I can control anger and hostility.	1	2	3	4

continue…

19. I have a network of friends doing social activities that I do.	1	2	3	4
20. I take time off to have some fun at least once a week	1	2	3	4
21. I am religious and this guides me and strengthens me.	1	2	3	4
22. I often provide service to others.	1	2	3	4
23. I enjoy my job/career.	1	2	3	4
24. I get along with coworkers/students.	1	2	3	4
25. I am a competent worker.	1	2	3	4
26. My income is sufficient for my needs.	1	2	3	4
27. I manage time properly.	1	2	3	4
28. I can say 'no' to additional load.	1	2	3	4
29. I take quiet time for myself every day.	1	2	3	4
30. I practice stress management as and when needed.	1	2	3	4

0 – 30 points – *Excellent (great resistance to stress)*

31–40 – *Good (little vulnerability to stress)*

41–50 – *Average (somewhat vulnerable to stress)*

51–60 – *Fair (vulnerable to stress)*

≥ 60 – Poor (highly vulnerable to stress)

Sometimes, we can change the situation or avoid stressors (stress-causing factors) but many times we cannot avoid them. For instance, due to a major illness of any close relative. Nevertheless, we can manage stress through relaxation techniques and time management. If you cannot manage time properly, you may experience chronic stress, fatigue, discouragement and illness.

Everybody wishes they had more time for exercise, recreation, hobbies and families. Healthy and successful people are good time managers and are able to maintain a pace of life, within their comfort zone. You have to learn to plan, scrutinize, eliminate unwanted wastage of time, add requisite activities, decide the priorities, set goals, achieve them, re-plan if necessary, get your tasks done, and reward yourself. You can thus manage the time, which is at your disposal. It can be done in such a way that the effect will help you manage stressors effectively.

Relaxation Techniques

Stress management skills are essential to cope with life effectively and move forward in today's fast-paced world. Although you may reap the benefits immediately after engaging in any of the several relaxation techniques, you need to practice them continuously to master them.

Let us learn the simple technique to manage stress.

Exercise: With exercise, you can reduce muscular tension and eliminate physiological changes that have triggered the fight or flight mechanism.

Physical exercise gives an overall boost by:

- lessening feelings of anxiety, depression, frustration, aggression, anger and hostility.

- alleviating insomnia.

- developing in you a desire to meet social needs and develop new friendships.

- developing in you a desire to share common interests and problems with others.

- helping you develop self-discipline.

- improving health and creating a sense of wellbeing.

The first important aspect of a healthy lifestyle is to lose your extra weight and maintain it. Exercise will help you do this. Take care to see that you are not making it compulsive and it is not becoming a stressor by itself. Exercising at your own pace causes secretion of happy hormones like endorphin, which gives the best relaxed feeling. Manage time and reserve one hour for scientific exercise.

Progressive Muscle Relaxation

In this technique, you are supposed to tighten and relax your muscles progressively, so that muscle tension is released and your body relaxes at will. You are supposed to practice this technique in a quiet, warm and well-ventilated room. You must tense the muscles one by one, by contracting them. You have to hold the contracted muscle for 5 seconds. Then relax it till it becomes totally limp. Follow this sequence from toe to top. A total of 20 minutes is required to perform this sequence for all the muscle groups, one after another. If you cannot invest this much of time at a stretch, you may divide it into three sessions, giving special attention to specific areas that are feeling very tense. First, stretch out comfortably on the floor, face up. Take a pillow under your knees. Assume a passive attitude and allow the body to relax as much as possible. Then, without any strain, contract each muscle group in sequence. Tighten each muscle group to only about 70% of the total muscle tension to avoid possible cramping. To produce the relaxation effects, pay attention to the sensation of tensing up and relaxing. Completing the entire sequence at one go yields the best results.

Breathing Techniques

In India, breathing exercises have been practiced since time immemorial to improve mental, physical and emotional stamina. In this, one must try to breathe away the tension and inhale fresh air and energy for the entire body. These exercises should be done in a quiet, pleasant, well-ventilated room, like any other relaxation technique.

Learn these simple breathing exercises as an antidote for stress.

Deep Breathing

Lie with your back flat on the floor. Place a pillow under your knees, separate the feet slightly with your toes pointing outward. (You can sit or stand straight up to perform this exercise). Place one hand on your abdomen and the other on your chest. Breathe in and out slowly, so that the hand on your abdomen rises when you inhale and falls as you exhale. The hand on your chest should not move at all. Repeat the exercise for about 10 times. Now, scan your body for possible tension and compare the present tension level with the tension level at the beginning.

* **Sighing** using the abdominal breathing techniques: Breathe in through your nose to a specific count, such as 4, 5, 6. Then exhale through pursed lips to double the intake count, such as 8, 10, 12. Repeat this 8 to 10 times when you are stressed.

* **Complete natural breathing:** Sit in an upright position or stand straight up. Breathe in through your nose, fill your lungs gradually from bottoms up. Hold your breath for several seconds. Now exhale slowly by allowing your chest and abdomen to relax completely. Repeat the exercise 8 to 10 times.

Meditation

The best way of relaxation and alleviation of the harmful physiological effects of stress is meditation. Meditate in a comfortable, quiet and disturbance-free-room, approximately for 15 minutes, twice a day. This will give you great pleasure.

- Sit in a chair in an upright position with your hands resting in your lap or on the arms of a chair. Close your eyes and focus on your breathing. Allow your body to relax as much as possible. Feel relaxed and watch your breathing.

- Allow your body to breathe regularly at its own rhythm.

- Repeat, in your mind, the word 'one,' every time you inhale and the word 'two' every time you exhale. Pay attention to these ones and twos and keep distressing thoughts from entering your mind.

- Continue this for about 15 minutes.

Concentrate on the midpoint between the eyebrows. Concentrate on the rhythm of pulse, any mantra, a pleasant memory or the wonders of nature like the rising sun or blooming flower. You may choose any event with which happy memories are associated. You can concentrate on your dream of a slim and fit figure too. The enchanting mantra of 'om,' any prayer or God's name can also help you meditate.

Try to live every moment of life with 100% participation in that moment. If you are reading, concentrate by giving 100%, if you are dancing, forget every other thing and give your 100% to the act of. Live every moment of life to its fullest potential. Then perhaps you may not need any other technique to relax.

If you learn to be diligent and start taking control of yourself, you will find that you can enjoy a better, happier and healthier life. All disorders cannot be cured through stress management and therapy. If they have not been effective for total cure, then you have to take the help of more specialized resources.

Chapter 12

Positive Mental Attitude

Think Positive, Be Positive

All efforts toward health, weight reduction and weight loss will give you 100% results if you think positively. Your positive mental attitude is an extremely crucial aspect for 100% success in anything that you attempt.

Positive thoughts: I know, I am overweight. I am aware that, besides my eating habits and other habits, so many other factors are involved in me being overweight. I want to lose weight. I am learning and following the correct method for it. I am committing myself to the healthy lifestyle prescribed in this book. I am doing this for my health. Even though I am late to start, it is better to be late than never. I will give my 100%, to change my lifestyle, even though results may fluctuate because of various controllable and uncontrollable reasons. I know the changes happening in my body are positive. I am better than yesterday and I will be still better tomorrow. Tomorrow, I will be better than today.

I am a responsible citizen and my juniors follow my example. So, it is my responsibility to give them a good message through my behavior. I am feeling better with this new lifestyle and I do not even think about my old wrong habits. I am lucky to know the way to good health. I am enjoying life better. I am very confident that I will definitely achieve my ideal weight.

Such thoughts, during your crucial period of weight reduction, help you travel steadily toward your goal. Your weight loss and maintenance will become easy and enjoyable. Your overall health will improve and you will realize that everything is happening positively due to positive thinking. Remember you can lose your extra weight efficiently when you are happy. Be positive and get a positive life. This lifestyle management program will give you a healthy life. Slowly and steadily, you enter an upbeat mood. Life becomes wonderful for you. You start living to its fullest potential. The changed lifestyle is now your normal lifestyle. You do not have to undertake additional pain to modify anything. Even if you miss your exercise for one day, you will feel that you are missing something pleasant and you will rush to do it immediately. When you see junk food, you will realize that it's junk and it's not for you. Your life will not be stressful and you will get an urge from within to do something for others, for society, for nature, for the environment. You would like to do something creative. You will create a great new personality, which is markedly different from your stale old persona. So, all the best. Wish you the best of health!

Chapter 13

Weight Maintenance

Introduction

Maintaining the reduced weight is more difficult if the weight has been lost by any other treatment than the ones prescribed in this book. Learn how to maintain and enjoy a healthy, slim and beautiful body forever!

If weight loss has been achieved through lifestyle management, you do not carry a huge risk of relapse or recurrence of weight gain, unless there is a break or gap in exercise, due to trauma, a major illness or pregnancy. In such cases, you have to control the calorie intake accordingly and resume exercise as soon as possible again, when you overcome the illness.

Even in normal conditions, you have to take care so that you maintain the reduced weight. Many times, you feel that you are slim, trim and fit like your friends and can indulge once in a while. When you meet your friends, you may get tempted to eat the food that is high in calories, which your friends are eating. Such a slip, once in a while, does not show any major change in your weight. Then you get the wrong idea that your body is now allowing you to eat like others. But if you lose control, you tend to indulge often, which leads to immediate weight gain.

We discussed earlier that emptied fat cells are unhappy, hungry cells and they grab the fats fast. This leads to more fat accumulation than before. Many times, you attend a party and eat something wrong. The next day, you try to compensate for it in your workout, by investing two extra hours in exercise. Then it becomes punishing for your body and mind. After losing the extra kilo you gained, you tend to skip the exercise. This rest after overexertion makes you feel good. Then the number of episodes of rest increase. Slowly, you move away from a healthy lifestyle. Then you start feeling guilty. Your weight may start going up again. Your friends remark that this often happens with a weight-loss program and you tend to put on more weight than before.

What Is the Solution?

You have to remember that your so-called slim friends are genetically slim. They have not struggled to become slim. You have achieved your weight loss after accepting extremely difficult changes in your lifestyle. Remember this new lifestyle has immense benefits.

Your friends may eat high-calorie food and it may not show up as immediate weight gain in their bodies as their metabolism is high. Your metabolism and your physiology will not allow you any additional calories often. Once in a while, it is fine. If you eat something you shouldn't eat, once in a while, there may not be any major change in weight. Even if there is a slight weight gain, it will come down in 3 to 4 days. It is not necessary to punish yourself by compensating through a heavy over workout.

In the last part of this book, there is an Appendix that shows the calories in specific food substances. Gain knowledge of it. Avoid junk food and empty calories. Even if you have shown no gain after consuming such food, do not practice this bad habit again and again.

The diet, as per your healthy lifestyle plan, is extremely nutritious and balanced. You can try the new low-cal recipes suggested in the Appendix. You have to change the patterns of a wrong lifestyle. You may also offer these suggestions to your friends, so that together we can prevent the chronic disorders in society, in this generation and the next. The food served in parties is not good even for slim people. Let us take the initiative to change the menu in parties so that everybody benefits. We have to remember that we have committed ourselves to a healthy lifestyle forever—for our good health and that of the next generation as well.

Chapter 14

Approaches to Be Avoided during Weight Reduction

Introduction

We have decided to lose weight for health. We have to follow a healthy lifestyle. During the weight-reduction program, we have to follow the principle that health is the prima facie of life and weight loss and beauty are the byproducts. To achieve this, the treatment must be safe and scientific.

You may get tempted by various advertisements that promise that you will lose 10 kg in 25 days. Many ads promote weight reduction without gym exercise, weight reduction with miracle supplements or fad diets. These types of treatment are scientifically wrong, have temporary results, and lead to serious health hazards later. Weight loss then remains a dream. It becomes more difficult to lose weight after the setback of 'miracle' treatments. What's worse, your health and body composition deteriorate. So, let us learn what we should not do for losing weight to get rid of obesity.

Many overweight and obese people try any number of approaches for weight loss, which are neither safe nor effective. It is very important to be aware of these methods and how they do or do not work.

- **Fad diets:** With a burning desire to lose weight quickly and easily, many obese people try fad diets. In such diets, only one type of food is recommended to be consumed. For example, Atkins diet recommends a high-protein and high-fat diet without restriction but it avoids carbohydrates, fruits, vegetables, and sugar in the diet. No sugar means no insulin; then the body starts breaking down fats. This leads to formation of Kenton bodies, which tend to reduce the appetite. Protein and fat help you feel full, but you do not get fibers and micronutrients. This diet may raise blood cholesterol. You lose weight at an extremely fast rate. But when you come back to the normal diet, there is a weight gain immediately. This sets up a yo-yo effect or weight cycling, along with nutritional deficiencies, cellular stress and other side effects.

GM diet recommends eating fruits the first day, vegetables the next day, followed by only proteins for the next two days. This leads to quick weight loss due to difficulty in eating the same food in one day in large quantities. However, you quickly become malnourished, pale and tired. You may lose 3–4 kg in a week but once you stop following this diet, you may gain 4–5 kg immediately. You may become heavier than what you were before starting the diet plan. The same scenario happens with Mayo diet, which recommends loading of only eggs and vegetables and no carbohydrates or fats. Beverly diet recommends only fruits.

Keto diet suggests you eat only fats and proteins. One gets deficiencies because of absence of complex carbohydrates. On top of that, when you resume your original diet, you will start to regain the weight again. At the same time, lipid profile shows increased cholesterol values, which are hazardous to health.

Intermittent diet allows you to have foo only twice a day with one long window. It is very difficult to fast for 16 or more hours. It may lead to hypoglycemia or acidity like troubles.

If you want to lose weight and maintain the weight loss, you have to get used to the idea that speed is not compatible with durability. It is better to lose at the rate of one kg per ten days, while adhering to good eating habits, than to lose a large amount of weight in a few days, only to put on all the weight and more later. Early and rapid weight loss is due to loss of glycogen in the kidneys, liver and muscle and protein breakdowns with large water loss. After 3–4 weeks, the rate of weight loss slows down.

Fad diets must be avoided at any cost. If you lose it quickly, you put on quickly. When it comes to slimming, durability is not compatible with speed. Be slow and steady and win the race.

Fasting: Fasting or starvation is clearly not a healthy way to lose weight. Fasting can lead to huge weight but as much as 60% of weight loss comes from lean mass, which is an undesirable outcome. Fasting has also been reported to cause severe degenerative changes in the heart muscle. Health and energy are also lost as the metabolism slows and electrolyte imbalances occur. The weight loss achieved during the fasting period is typically regained quickly. When you regain the weight, you regain fats or adipose tissue and the lost muscles are not obtained back immediately. Your body composition is worse than before. You have more fats and fewer muscles than before. Now, even if you eat lesser than before, you cannot burn the calories at the rate at which you were burning them before. Instead, you start gaining more and more weight.

Results That Show More Weight Than Before

Our primary concern is to stay fit and energetic and be immune to diseases.

Diet and No Exercise

Dieting means taking less amount of energy than your body expends. The body first burns whatever carbohydrates it has, then it burns proteins from your muscle tissue and some fats. So, in 4 weeks, if you lose 4 kg, your actual weight loss would be as follows:

40% fat loss + 60% muscle loss

	Before	Loss	After dieting
Weight	80 kg	– 4 kg	76 kg
% Fat	35%	—	34.73%
Fat weight	28 kg	– 1.6 kg	26.4 kg
LBM	52 kg	– 2.4 kg	49.6 kg

You have lost 1.6 kg of fat. That is not much of fat loss. The major change has occurred in your LBM. You have actually lost 2.4 kg of muscles. Loss of muscle means loss of strength and loss of energy. Your ability to sustain any kind of exercise goes down. You get tired all the time. Your body's metabolism and capacity to burn calories have reduced. If your body needed 1500 calories before, it may now need only 1300 calories.

You start looking tired and haggard and feel drained out. So, you go off the diet and start eating your usual high-fat meals. It gives you quick satisfaction. But now you are feeding your body extra calories when it needs less, as your LBM is down. The excess calories are more than before. Your body quickly turns all that 'excess' into fat. As you don't exercise, all the weight gained consists of fat alone. You are back to having a body weight of 80 kg. Now look at the negatively changed body composition.

	Before	After dieting (4 weeks later)	Off diet (8 weeks later)
Weight	80 kg	76 kg	80 kg
% Fat	35%	34.73%	38%
Fat weight	28 kg	26.4 kg	30.4 kg
LBM	52 kg	49.6 kg	49.6 kg

Even though you weigh the same as before, you are now fatter than before and have less LBM. Your energy level and stamina have reduced. You are worse than what you started with.

Now, let us look at a specific example of how exercise, with proper diet control, promotes fat loss.

Participant : Male

Age : 36 years

Diet : No fats, no sweets, no fried food

Height : 5ft. 10 in Healthy eating

Exercise schedule : 3 days bench workouts (1 hour each) + 3 days training with weights (1 hour each)

	Before	After 6 weeks	Net change
Weight	79 kg	78 kg	– 1 kg
Fat%	36.6%	30%	– 6.6%
Fat weight	25.3 kg	20.4 kg	– 4.9 kg
LBM	43.7 kg	47.6 kg	+ 3.9 kg
Lower abdomen	42.5"	37"	– 5.5"

The participant has lost fat around the arms, abdomen and thighs—a loss of approximately 5 kg. In the process, he has firmed up his body. He has gained strength, which is reflected in his increased LBM of almost 4 kg. All tests of strength and endurance have shown tremendous improvement. Earlier, he could not do a single push up, he can now do 18. If you practice the same type of routine, then your energy improves and your stamina increases. Your self-confidence increases, so does your commitment to good eating and exercise. Thus, you continue the process of further fat loss and fulfill the quest for an attractive body shape. A gradual weight loss of ½–1 kg/week is the best way to lose ½ kg of fat. You need to burn 3500 calories to lose ½ kg of fat.

Crash diets are harmful because they:

- slow the body's metabolism.

- burn muscles for energy.

- conserve fat.

- set you up for binging.

Weight-loss drugs are ineffective. They are risky and may have some side effects.

The body resists rapid change, so one must lose weight gradually. So, healthy weight loss is brought about by **eating right + exercises + sensible lifestyle habits,** combined with **desire + determination + consistency.**

Very Low-Calorie Diets (VLCD)

VLCDs have been used many times as a last resort for seriously obese people. Consumption of several liquid meals throughout the day containing 800 kcal/day together is the characteristic feature of VLCD. These meals contain high proteins to attenuate the loss of lean tissue and 100% RDA of essential vitamins and minerals. It is important to emphasize that VLCD can only be used when the dieter is under the care and supervision of a physician. Interestingly, a person who follows VLCD experiences significant decrease in hunger and shows interest in food after one or two weeks. If this treatment is followed with behavior modifications, a weight-maintenance program, and most importantly under the continuous supervision of a physician, it is found to be useful. Still it is not advisable for adults, pregnant and lactating mothers, and elderly people with psychiatric disorders. The failure to continue leads to weight gain, again and again.

In this book, we are repeatedly learning the message and educating ourselves that a combination of a balanced nutritious low-cal diet, a scientific exercise regime and acceptance of changes in our lifestyle forever is the only magic solution for weight reduction and weight maintenance.

Chapter 15

Prevention of Obesity

Introduction

Prevention of an ounce is equal to cure of a pound! Only if we will prevent these lifethreatening disorders in time, can we keep them away and enjoy good health. For that, we have to educate ourselves and manage our lifestyle during pregnancy and manage the lifestyle of our children in early childhood and in adolescence. If we can provide our next generation with scientific education about obesity, by inculcating good habits since their childhood, we can prevent obesity as well as health risks associated with obesity.

For prevention of risky health hazards and promotion of health, to build a strong and healthy new generation, let us learn this chapter carefully.

It is a well-known fact that Indians have more fat percentage. The legacy of Indian bodies is to store than to utilize. We have to change this tendency. We must do this not only for ourselves but also for posterity, even though this may take years to achieve.

A. Nutrition Awareness

- A child should be taught nutrition thoroughly. We have to inculcate good nutritious eating habits right from his or her childhood. A balanced diet includes complex carbohydrates, seasonal fresh fruits and vegetables, fiber-rich food, limited simple carbohydrates, recommended quantities of lean proteins, limited fats and lots of water.

- Junk food like bakery products, biscuits, chocolates, chips, pizzas, burgers, fried food, instant noodles, sweets, ice creams, pastries, refined products, soft drinks, juices of fruits instead of fruits, milkshakes, puddings and ready-to-eat instant products should be kept away from the child after educating him or her about nutrition.

- Feeding children with wrong food in the wrong quantity does not prove your love to them. On the contrary, such love will be responsible for their bad health in future. It is your responsibility to inculcate the following good habits in your child:

> ➤ Have a good fresh breakfast, preferably prepared at home.

> ➤ Eat in small quantities and eat frequently.

> ➤ Eat at one place, preferably sitting at the dining table.

> ➤ Eat slightly less.

> ➤ Eat by chewing food.

> ➤ Drink lots of water.

> ➤ Strictly avoid food in front of the TV.

> ➤ Avoid junk food.

> ➤ Include maximum fruits and vegetables. Celebrate without high-calorie junk food. Celebrate with nutritious, limited homemade good food.

> ➤ Count the calories.

> ➤ Always think about the nutrition and always keep in mind whether it is necessary to eat just now.

- Plan the food intake, preferably taking the help of a dietician, and update it from time to time, if possible.

- Learn recommended dietary allowances and teach them to your child.

- Prefer natural sources of food than preserved foods.

  > ➤ Avoid heavy dinner late at night.

- Pick the role models whom the child adores and try to find out their food habits.

- Praying before the meal and having peace of mind and a pleasant atmosphere at dining table will help the child build a good psychology.

- Teach a child the habit of solving problems with discussion and overcoming stress with proper management instead of overeating to feel relaxed.

- Do not drink alcohol or smoke in front of the child.

B. Exercise

Try to make a child physically active. Let the child use the staircase, encourage him or her to walk small distances. Teach the child cycling and swimming. Encourage him or her to participate in outdoor games, trekking and skill games. Let the child join NCC, do yoga or dance. Make sure the child is active throughout the day and is spending at least one hour in an activity that makes him or her sweat a lot. If one of the parents or both parents are obese, then make sure the child is engaged in a physical activity, which will help him or her build strong musculature and improve BMR. Athlete training, gymnastics, martial arts and horse riding are some of the options. Participating in such activities helps change the body composition.

Discourage the child from opting for sedentary activities like video games and computers. Spend a holiday in a repair workshop or a garage. Go for long walks, trekking, swimming with your child, instead of going to the movies. Make your child be friendly with nature. Try to convert your child's body into a calorie-burning machine. A child who exercises can concentrate better in studies than the child who watches TV. The child who exercises becomes stronger, flexible, fit and can cope up with any physical or psychological situation. Children engaged in sports have a sporty nature and face the problems of life in a sporty way. In a healthy and fit body, there is always a healthy, cheerful and creative mind. Do not let children be a part of a rat race. Do not let them lose health and fitness for a career. For a better future, health and fitness, along with a good career, are equally important.

C. Effects of Exercise on Fat Cells

Exercise in Young Age

Exercise in young age attenuates the rate of proliferation of fat cells. Entering adulthood with fewer fat cells will help an individual reduce his chances of becoming an overweight adult. Even in adulthood, the size of fat cells reduces due to exercise but the number of adipocytes does not reduce. This speaks of the need to exercise in an early age for prevention of obesity.

D. After menarche (starting of monthly period), take care that your girl is getting scientific training about body composition to keep the fat percentage in the right balance. Give her a clear idea about the reasons for obesity and your plan to train her for maintaining her fat and her future child's fat percentage under control by committing to a healthy lifestyle. Concentrate on strengthening LBM.

Remember, girls will never build muscles like boys as the female hormones will not allow them to do so, even if they wish to (unless they take male hormones externally).

E. Education Before and during Pregnancy

Generally, women develop health awareness only during pregnancy. They have to be educated even before. Let women read pregnancy fitness books, learn prenatal exercises, and learn more about nutrition and supplements. Do not overfeed your girl child because your parents overfed you. Do not make her rest unless she is advised to do so. The advice of the gynecologist, dietician and health expert should be taken and followed meticulously. This will save her from obesity and her child will get proper health education in the womb itself. This will be helpful for the child's body composition.

F. Breastfeeding

Breastfeeding a child is like an insurance policy against obesity. This has been proven to be a scientific fact.

G. First Year in an Infant's Life

Many people think that a fat and chubby baby is a healthy baby. This is a very wrong notion. Generally, the number of fat cells a person would have is decided in the first year itself. Thereafter, the size increases. If we can restrict this number, through proper diet, then the fat percentage will not exceed and the chances of developing obesity can be minimized. The infant will be grateful to you forever if you restrict the number of fat cells in its body.

H. Control of Carbohydrate Intake during the First Year

It is an undisputed fact that a large intake of carbohydrates plays a crucial role in causing obesity. In the present scenario, weaning a child during the third month of its life is common as mothers are working women. In such cases, do not feed child carbohydrates. Do not add sugar to milk. Instead, try a balanced diet after consulting a doctor. Try to avoid carbohydrate addiction. A balanced diet is very important. Try to continue breastfeeding till the ninth month.

I. Chewing Is Very Important

Train the child to use the teeth properly. Food that does not need chewing should be avoided. Do not provide soft foods that can be swallowed easily. Let the child chew and make the food soft, so that he or she can swallow the same easily.

J. Create a Proper Environment for the Child

Let the child feel safe and secure in the house. Let him or her not be deprived of parental attention and affection. Otherwise, the child may start relying on food to feel safe and secure. He or she will compensate for the lack of love through overeating. It is your duty to fulfill the psychological needs of children. Love, warmth and compassion make the child happy. For the betterment of the child, you have to nurture and maintain an atmosphere of mutual goodwill in your home.

K. Start educating your child about the aspects of a healthy lifestyle as early as possible. Your commitment to a healthy lifestyle should work as an example for your child to follow.

Chapter 16

F.A Q.s. (Frequently Asked Questions)

Q1. I want to lose my tummy alone. I do not want to lose my upper body at all. Should I do only more and more sit-ups? Should I avoid exercises for the upper body?

Answer: Reduction and maintenance of measurements in abdomen needs a four-fold treatment.

- You have to increase your calorie expenditure. For this, you have to do aerobics workout at least three days a week. With aerobic exercise, you have to burn fats. Take care that intensity, duration and frequency are as recommended.

- You have to control intake of calories. High-fat food is to be avoided strictly. Total calorie intake should be restricted. Diet prescribed in healthy lifestyle is to be consumed.

- You have to do gym exercises to increase your metabolism rate. Your lean body mass gets stronger. Your calorie-burning capacity goes up, and this leads to utilization of calories instead of them getting stored in the form of fats.

Important note: Only abdominal exercises do not cause reduction in measurements. Exercises make the muscles stronger and toned. To burn the fats around the abdominal region, the three aspects of aerobics training, calorie control and gym training are most important.

Spot reduction is a myth. If, by working the same part again and again, one can lose the measurements of that part, then all tennis players would have a very slim fore arm of the right or left hand, whichever hand they use at least for 3–4 hours every day. However, exercising the same part again and again leads to training of that muscle; the strength and endurance of that muscle increases. This improves toning and may lead to better appearance than before. This is the spot training effect.

Using belts, ointments or any pack will not burn the fats on any part. The water from the cell gets utilized and thus temporary change in measurements is possible. But, once you stop the use of such passive treatment, then the tummy reappears; perhaps with increased measurements.

Word of caution:

- *Do not practice more than 4–5 sets of abdominal exercises every day. This gives undue stress on the spine in the lumber region.*

- *Do extension exercise of the lower back after abdominals. Yogasanas like Bhujangasana, Shalabhasan and twisting of the waist must be done (at least five times each) after abdominal exercises.*

- *Do not do neck movements or push the neck to contract abdominals while doing sit-ups. You have to contract the abdominals alone; concentrate on it so that, automatically, the upper body gets lifted up. Pushing the upper body with the hands behind the neck will not help contract the abdominals. Contracting the abdominal muscles leads to lifting of the shoulders and neck. The movement of the neck with each sit-up may lead to pain in the neck.*

- *Correct techniques of abdominal exercise are extremely necessary in order to isolate the muscle. The same is true for both the hips and thighs. Spot training is possible, while spot reduction is a myth.*

The upper body muscles are pectoralis muscles. You can increase the size of the pectoralis muscles with specific gym exercises. Good postures and big pectoral muscles will improve the measurements of the upper body. Female breasts are not muscle tissues. They are fats and milk glands. They cannot grow with any exercise. During pregnancy, after child birth and during menopause, the breasts show increased size because of hormonal changes. There is no any exercise or any cream that can increase the breast size in females.

Q2. Will I look like a man after doing gym exercises? Do women body builders do gym exercises to develop muscles like men?

Answer: Women do not develop muscles like men by doing gym exercises. Men have more muscle mass, greater capacity for muscle hypertrophy and an ability of the muscles to increase in size. This larger capacity of muscle hypertrophy is related to sex-specific hormones. Similarly, variations in the extent of masculinity and femininity are determined by individual differences in the hormonal secretions of androgen, testosterone, estrogens and progesterone.

The male hormone, testosterone, is responsible for muscle hypertrophy. For body building, very intense training for two or more hours, like constant weight lifting, with short intervals has to be performed. The weight lifted is at the maximum capacity of a person. After such training, with the effect of testosterone, the muscles show hypertrophy. Women neither have testosterone nor can they perform such a demanding workout. So, hypertrophy and size of muscles that can be achieved in males is next to impossible in women.

Women body builders use external anabolic steroids and human growth hormones. These hormones lead to muscular hypertrophy. Such drugs cause increased muscle size and side effects like hypertension, fluid retention, smaller breasts, hoarseness of voice and facial hair like men. Without such drugs, women cannot have muscle hypertrophy.

Gym exercises, on the contrary, are extremely useful for women as they lead to enhancement in strength, endurance, basal metabolism rate, lean mass, body composition and bone strength.

Gym exercises give good posture, good physique and a toned body. This is the reason why all leading women film stars and models do gym exercises.

Q3. Are strong muscles important to men only?

Answer: Muscles perform all physical activities in men as well as in women. Both have to meet the physical challenges as per their capacities. Each of us has the ability to develop more strength and muscle tone. Additionally, muscle-strengthening exercises strengthen bones and connective tissues as well. If we do not do gym exercises, we lose approximately ½ pound of muscle physiologically per year, after the age of 35. To prevent muscle loss and strengthen muscles, gym exercises are vital for both men and women.

Q4. Is aerobics (running/swimming/aerobic classes) more important to lose weight than gym exercises?

Answer: Participating in an aerobics class three times a week is good for your health. It burns 400 kcal per session but it does not boost your metabolism for 24 hours a day. If you increase your lean body mass by doing a gym workout, then your BMR is boosted. Gym exercises have a residual effect for the next 24 hours (till the next session of exercise), which burns calories for all 24 hours. Whereas, aerobic exercise burns fats only for 1 hour; TEE (thermic effect of exercise) of aerobics lasts for 2–3 hours. Wear and tear of muscle tissue goes on for 24–48 hours. There are more than 600 muscles in the body. If you do not make them stronger and balanced, then they get weaker slowly. This leads to reduction in metabolism. During aerobics, due to overweight, joints like knee, hips and in the spine (weight bearing joints) get exerted to a large extent. It is always beneficial to perform gym exercises one after another continuously to derive some benefits of aerobics and for total safety and effective weight reduction.

Q5. When one stops exercising, do muscles get 'turned into fat'?

Answer: Muscle cells and fat cells are completely different. One cannot turn into other. Muscles are made up of proteins while fats cells are depots of fats alone. When you stop calorie output, your muscles get weaker. Energy balance gets disturbed. Stopping exercises stops expending 400 to 500 kcal per day. This leads to storage of fats. The fat percentage increases due to stoppage of calorie burning. No muscle gets turned into fats.

Q6. If I stop aerobics, will I become obese again immediately?

Answer: If you discontinue any exercise, you stop calorie burning through that exercise. It may be aerobic or gym exercise or plain walking. Your energy balance gets disturbed and you start putting on weight again. You have to do some sort of exercise throughout life and become physically active. Exercise is an important aspect of a healthy lifestyle.

Q7. Does heavy sweating during exercise help a person lose fat?

Answer: Sweating is water loss. If you do not replace water regularly, then you may get dehydrated. The loss of water due to dehydration varies from 1 to 4 liters from person to person. Once you replace the fluid, you show the previous weight. Even if you do not sweat during exercise of one hour or sweat less than another person, you approximately burn the equivalent calories for the same exercise of the same intensity and type. (Some difference due to weight difference and intensity variation is possible.)

Sweating is water loss, not fat loss. However, fluid replacement is crucial for optimal performance and proper heat balance.

Q8. Are steam baths, sauna baths effective in weight loss?

Answer: No. The weight loss due to steam or sauna is water loss. If you have steam or sauna and immediately stand on a scale, it will show a great difference in weight, which is due to water loss. As soon as you replace the water, you gain the lost water weight.

Steam bath and sauna bath are the best modes of relaxation. Due to the hot atmosphere, the pores open up, blood circulation gets diverted to the skin, and blood vessels are dilated. Toxins get excreted through the open pores. The brain releases the happy hormone, endorphin, and you feel relaxed. A chilled bath, followed by steam, causes immediate constriction of the peripheral blood vessels and the tightening of skin and pores. This improves skin toning. Though steam and sauna are the best modes of relaxation, they have nothing to do with weight loss. Even passive modes like vibrating belts, rollers, tummy belts, corsets, ointments, pills and massages do not help lose weight. Fat cannot be 'shaken off'; the body has to use it as an energy substrate. Fat is lost efficiently by burning it in the muscle tissue.

Section IV

Medical Aspects of Obesity

Introduction of Doctors Who Have Contributed in This Section

Status Health Club is a **medical** and **wellness club**. *We also have an associated wellness clinic for diagnosis. We have a panel of expert medical practitioners who are highly qualified and are keen in promoting of health in society. These medical experts are experiencing a healthy lifestyle by exercising in Status Health Club. They practice what they preach.*

We, at Status Health Club, believe in doing our share in building a healthy and fit community. Status Health Club is successfully running the 'Obesity Elimination Program' in association with an expert medical panel for creating awareness in society.

Dr. Sanjay Gupte *is the president of the panel. He is a role model for all of us as he exercises regularly and maintains his weight at an ideal level. He has been a member of Status Health Club from its inception. In this book, he enlightens us on obesity and PCOS.*

Dr. Vaishali and Dr. Parag Biniwale *are the young generation gynecologists who are talking about obesity, pregnancy and menopause.*

Dr. Lily Joshi *is a physician who is very active in the promotion of health and a healthy lifestyle. In this book, she has discussed obesity and certain medical conditions like diabetes type II.*

Dr. Anuradha Sowani *is an oncologist who is very active in her field, working as the chief consultant at CIPLA CANCER. In this book, she talks about the correlation between obesity and cancer.*

Dr. Jagdish Hiremath *is a leading cardiologist. He is very keen in the promotion of a healthy lifestyle in society. He practices the principles of Dean Aurnish for reversal of heart diseases. Dr. Hiremath has given information on obesity and cardiovascular diseases in this book.* **Dr. Sanika Mijjar** *is a co-contributor.*

Dr. Vaman Khadilkar *is an endocrinologist and has given information on obesity in adolescence. He is very keen on prevention of obesity in childhood and adolescence.*

Dr. Ashish Babhulakar *has pointed out the relationship between obesity and osteoarthritis.*

Dr. Sachin Tapsvi *has shown the relation between obesity and knee joint.*

Dr. Lily Joshi *has presented her thoughts on coping with obesity.*

The **'special population'** *with certain medical conditions needs special modifications in the exercise and nutrition program. After every chapter, I have presented some dos and don'ts, along with the required modifications for a healthy lifestyle.*

We have a unique opportunity at our fingertips. We have all the information collectively in a book form.

I am extremely proud to say I am the luckiest obesity practitioner to have such a valuable panel of experts, who are very enthusiastic to guide us and enlighten us about the prevention and cure of medical conditions associated with obesity and the promotion of health in society. I hope this book becomes the Gita or gospel to be referred to—for obesity treatment, for me as well as for all those who want to fight the demon of obesity.

I am extremely thankful and grateful to all the experts who have provided their valuable insights. I owe them a lot throughout my life.

I have incorporated a very few sample cases, out of more than 15,000 successfully-treated clients, in my long and fruitful career of 25 years. I owe my gratitude to all my clients, who are enjoying the benefits of a healthy lifestyle prescribed by me and are healthy and fit for a long duration of time. Get inspired by these cases. Get benefited by the knowledge provided by experts. Commit yourself to a healthy lifestyle. Be healthy and fit!

Chapter 17

Obesity and Cancer

Dr. Anuradha Sowani
M.D. (internal medicine)
Diploma Pal. Med. (UK)
Consultant Medical Oncologist
Medical Director, Cipla Cancer Palliative Care Centre, Pune

In India, occurrence of cancer is increasing day by day. About 60% of the total deaths are due to cancers and cardiovascular diseases. More than 100 types of cancers can develop in the body. Cancer cells grow for no reason and multiply, destroying normal tissue. If the spread of cells is not controlled, it results in death.

Maintaining the recommended body weight is extremely essential in prevention of some cancers. Obesity may be associated with cancers of colon, rectum, breast, uterus, endometrium, kidney and prostate. In obesity, fats get deposited initially beneath the skin. When the fat percentage increases, more and more additional fats get deposited all over the body, for instance, inside the lumen of blood vessels, around various organs, and in between and among muscle fibers. In these fat depots, other toxins, fractions of some medicines, drugs and hormones get deposited.

As we have discussed in the chapter on nutrition, during metabolism, most of the oxygen in the human body is utilized for energy formation. During this process, carbon dioxide and water are also produced. However, many times free radicals are formed.

Carcinogenic substances like nicotine, alcohol, pollutants, oxygen-free radicals and other toxins deposited in fat depots, like some drugs and some traces of hormones, attack the normal cell membrane and DNA, leading to the formation of cancers.

Cell growth is controlled by DNA and RNA. When the carcinogenic substances mentioned above attack the cell walls and DNA, the cell loses its ability to regulate and control cell growth. Cell division is disturbed and cells grow uncontrollably and abnormally, forming a mass of tissue called 'tumor.' This tumor can get malignant. The tumor may go on for months and years without any significant growth. To grow, tumor requires more oxygen and nutrients. In time, a few cancer cells break away from the malignant tumor and migrate to other parts where they cause new cancer. Once it starts spreading, then it becomes difficult to control it. The good news is that cancer is largely preventable. As much as 80% of cancer is related to lifestyle or environmental factors like obesity, faulty diet, tobacco, alcohol, pollution, sexual and reproductive activities and stress. Lifestyle management through a healthy lifestyle is an effective way to prevent cancers.

Prevention of Cancer

Guidelines

Education is necessary about risk factors and lifestyle management through a healthy lifestyle.

Exercise (physical activity): An active lifestyle seems to have protective effects against cancer. Physical fitness and cancer have a consistent inverse relationship. Daily exercise of 50 minutes with moderate intensity lowers the risk of colon cancer, breast cancer and reproductive system cancer, by 20% to 30%. Moderate exercise improves the auto-immune system. The auto-immune system may play a role in preventing cancer. Yet the exact mechanism is not clear.

Dietary changes: A healthy diet is crucial to decrease the risk of cancer.

The diet should:

- be high in fiber and low in fat.

- contain fiber-rich vegetables, soy products, calcium and omega three fatty acids.

- have a protein intake, as per RDA.

- have no tobacco or alcohol.

- have obesity control.

Antioxidants absorb free radical phytochemicals found abundantly in all vegetables and fruits, described under 'protective food' in the chapter on nutrition.

They help:

- remove carcinogens from cells before they cause damage.

- activate enzymes that destroy cancer-causing-agents.

- prevent carcinogens from locking onto cells.

- prevent carcinogens from binding to the DNA.

- prevent cancer-causing precursors from being formed.

Fat-rich food increases bile secretion. Interaction of bile acids with intestinal bacteria releases carcinogenic byproducts.

Daily consumption of 25 to 35 gm (six to eight servings of vegetables or fruits) of fiber is very useful. Fiber binds to the bile in the intestine for excretion from the body through stools. Fiber-rich vegetables, fruits and grains also provide vitamins, minerals like folate selenium and calcium. These are helpful in protection from many cancers. Epigallocathechin (EGCC) found in green vegetables and green tea is a cancer-fighting agent.

Fat intake should be restricted and monounsaturated fats and omega three fatty acids are to be incorporated. Protein should not exceed RDA. Grilling meat on a high temperature for a long time increases carcinogenic substances on the surface of the meat. Soy protein helps in prevention of cancer they contain chemicals that prevent cancers. Phyto-chemicals found in soy protein are similar to estrogens and they help in prevention of spread of cancer. Giving up consumption of alcohol and smoking are very important steps in prevention of cancer.

The recommended body weight should be maintained. The treatment for prevention of cancer and treatment for obesity, described in this book, are similar.

Abstaining from Cigarettes

Cigarette smoking itself is a major health illness. The World Health Organization estimates that smoking causes 3 million deaths worldwide annually. The average life expectancy for a chronic smoker is about 15 years less than a non-smoker. About 87% of lung cancers are connected to smoking and 28% of all cancers are connected to smoking. Smoking should be stopped immediately.

Other Cancer-Causing Reasons

Exposure to ultraviolet radiations through sun, intake of estrogens (hormonal replacement therapy), X-ray exposure and occupational hazards are other reasons for cancer and must be avoided. Eating fried food, which is not cooked in the house, wherein the same oil and pans are used again and again, leads to the formation of carcinogenic substances. Such food should be strictly avoided.

Many cancers can be cured through early detection. Regular check-up will help detect cancer. Prevention is always better than cure. Food processing agents, artificial colors, saccharine, pesticides and high level of mental stress are to be avoided along with a change in lifestyle.

Lifestyle management through a healthy lifestyle is the solution for prevention. It is described in this book in an extremely methodical way. I am thankful to Dr. Sumedha for helping lay persons be aware of scientific exercises in the weight reduction program and the need for a nutritious balanced diet. Most importantly, she has compiled detailed information about antioxidant food sources, protective foods against cancer and stress management techniques, in this book.

The healthy lifestyle described in the book is not only helpful to lose weight and maintain it but will also help you keep away from cancer and other chronic disorders.

Change your lifestyle and enjoy a quality life! Follow the treatment and enjoy a slim body and healthy life!

Chapter 18

Obesity, Diabetes and Other Medical Conditions

Dr. Lily Joshi
M.D. (medicine)

India is poised to have many things. Some are good, some are bad, some are even disasters. While rural India is still struggling to overcome extreme poverty and malnutrition, the fast-expanding urban India is facing another kind of malnutrition that only affluence can bring in, resulting in obesity.

Obesity is widely prevalent in all our metro cities and is now spreading to smaller cities and towns with astonishing speed. Obesity is much more than a cosmetic concern. Anyone who is obese does not look good but also does not feel good. This is because obesity exposes a person to several health hazards that affect all the systems of the body. In that sense, obesity is a multi-system disorder.

In Section I, we learned in detail about obesity, its measurements, its diagnosis, and its causes. Why are we so concerned about obesity? Is it simply because we hate to look fat? Actually, fat beneath the skin, double chin, rolls on the back and the sides, and bulging thighs are all examples of subcutaneous fats, which are harmless. In fact, having fat thighs may be an advantage according to some studies. Then who is culprit of all complications? It is the visceral fat—the fat that lies within the internal organs and around the internal organs like liver, pancreas, kidneys, bowel loops and muscle fibers. This fat, rather than being an inert mass, behaves like an active endocrine organ. Like endocrinal glands, visceral fat generates many chemicals that work like hormones. These chemicals have deleterious effects on metabolism. This leads to diseased conditions. A person having lots of visceral fats generally stores it inside the abdominal cavity and hence the person is said to be centrally obese. Thus, central adiposity, rather than overall obesity, brings about a huge array of complications.

Let us discuss some complications of obesity in detail, which you must know how to manage for your good health.

Diabetes Mellitus

It is a chronic metabolic disorder due to diminished secretion of insulin by the pancreas (insulin is the hormone that promotes the entry of glucose into the body cells) or the inability of the body to utilize insulin. Diabetes mellitus leads to numerous health problems such as vision loss, circulatory problems like heart failure, kidney failure and nerve disorders, and death. Type II diabetes mellitus is the most common form of diabetes mellitus in 90% of diabetics. The main predisposing factor is obesity.

Fat induces insulin resistance. It does not allow the insulin secreted by pancreatic cells to be effective. Fats deposited around and within the pancreas hamper the sensitivity of insulin. There is inappropriate secretion of insulin. This leads to fatigue of the pancreas. Hence, the pancreas fails to perform its function effectively. Fats present around muscle fibers disturb the glucose consumption by the muscle. The uptake of glucose through muscles gets decreased. In liver, additional fats get deposited, they favor the breakdown of liver glycogen into glucose. The total effect of all these is an increase in blood glucose level and the presence of sugar in urine. Then diabetes is manifested.

Syndrome X

As the cells resist the action of insulin, the pancreas releases more insulin in an attempt to keep the blood level from rising. A chronic rise in insulin seems to trigger a series of abnormalities referred to as **syndrome X or metabolic syndrome.**

The abnormal conditions include low HDL, high triglycerides and increased blood clotting mechanism. Many individuals with syndrome X also have high blood pressure. All these conditions increase CHD and other diabetes related health conditions (like kidney failure, infection, blindness and nerve damage).

Currently, India has been declared the 'diabetes capital of the world.' This disease has been found even in the young population. A huge proportion of our population is getting affected by this serious multi-system disorder. Again, the solution for this disorder is lifestyle management through a healthy lifestyle.

Special Modifications in the Life Style Management Program for Diabetics

Dr. Sumedha Bhosale

Obesity is the predisposing factor for type II diabetes mellitus. Treatment of type II DM includes medication, change in diet, exercise and weight loss, if required.

Role of Exercise in Diabetes Control

It makes muscle cells more permeable to glucose, allowing the body to make better use of insulin. Utilization of glucose through the muscle cells improves because of exercise. Due to exercise, fat loss and weight loss happen, if calories are controlled. The risk of heart disease is also reduced.

Exercise Recommended

Low-intensity exercise for longer duration is useful for diabetics. Aerobic exercise for a minimum of 4–5 days a week with moderate intensity for 50 to 60 minutes per session, gym exercises on alternate days with low resistance and more repetitions and flexibility stretches every day, for 1 minute, followed by gym/aerobic session, are found to be extremely beneficial.

Special precautions to be taken:

- The patient must be educated about the signs and symptoms of hypoglycemia.

- The patient must discuss the exercise plan with the physician and insulin dosages must be re-planned accordingly.

- The timing of the exercise should be the same every day.

  ➢ Two hours prior to exercise, the patient should have a good breakfast. It is also necessary to have a drink or a fruit 30 minutes after the exercise session.

- The patient must carry rapid-acting carbohydrate, such as a packet of glucose, to correct hypoglycemia immediately, if it occurs.

- Insulin should not be injected in the muscle group, which is to be worked in that exercise session, so that it does not get absorbed at a faster rate. Otherwise, the patient may become hypoglycemic due to quick absorption of insulin.

- It is preferable to work with the instructor or partner after giving him/her idea about diabetes and symptoms of hypoglycemia.

- Exercise should be avoided during peak insulin activity.

- You must wear good footwear. Take good care of your feet by checking for cuts, blisters and signs of infection regularly.

- Exercise in excessive heat may exacerbate the risk of heat injuries with autonomic neuropathy.

- Friction of nylon clothes in the underarm area may cause skin rash, which may turn into infection. Therefore, avoid nylon clothing and friction. Use soft cotton garments during exercise. Use talcum powder at the sites of friction after exercise, after making the site clean and dry (under arms and waist u).

- Avoid exercise if there is retinopathy.

- Re-planning of the dosage of medication and timing of food should be done prior to starting exercise by the physician.

If you exercise with these precautions and follow the prescribed diet, you may have to stop the medication. Almost surely, you have to take only a nominal maintenance dose of oral medication. A healthy lifestyle prevents and manages diabetes. It definitely improves the quality of life of a diabetic patient.

Even a modest weight loss up to 10% is found to be extremely useful to improve glucose level and reduce the dosage of hypoglycemic medication. Syndrome X patients are also benefited from the weight-loss program. If one loses 8–9 kg of extra weight, there is a 40% drop in insulin resistance. About 45 minutes of exercise every day enhances insulin efficiency by 25%. Cessation of smoking too is extremely useful.

Other Medical Conditions of Obesity to Be Taken Care of Dr. Lily Joshi

- **Gall bladder disease:** Obesity is very closely linked to gall stones, which are usually made of fatty molecules. Gall stones can remain silent for many years, but when they cause obstruction to the flow of bile, complications like inflammation of gall bladder and pancreas may ensue, posing a serious threat to life.

- **Fatty liver disease:** Deposition of fat within and around the liver cells has been mentioned already. This directly impairs the liver function. People who suffer from this can develop serious problems later, though they remain symptom-free for a long time.

- **Abdominal and inguinal hernias:** Intermittent deposition of fat and lax abdominal muscles lead to weakening of the abdominal wall, through which the protrusions of inner organs take place. These are called hernias. Most of the times, these require surgical correction.

- **Varicose veins and deep vein thrombosis:** Obese women have an enlarged venous bed in the legs and suffer from leg edema (swelling in legs), heaviness and pain. At the same time, there are other complications like varicose eczemas, varicose ulcers and even deep vein thrombosis. **Deep vein thrombosis** is a potentially fatal condition if left untreated. It may lead to pulmonary embolism very rarely.

- **Skin disorders** like eczemas, ulcers and yellow deposits around the eyes called xanthelesma

- **Other conditions:** Blackish streaks of acanthesis nigricans are some conditions that go hand in hand with obesity. Excessive sweating, fungal infection and pyoderma are also common.

- **Neurosis** like anxiety, depression, lack of self-esteem, loss of confidence, eating disorders, sense of futility and frustrations are some common mood disorders found in obese people.

- Lastly, obese people tend to be **slow** and **clumsy** and hence **accident prone**. They sustain falls more commonly and are generally not able to support themselves to prevent accident.

My Views

Dr. Sumedha Bhosale

All conditions discussed above potentially affect the quality of life. Prevention of obesity is the best solution. A healthy lifestyle is the best way to prevent as well as to cure obesity and promote good health. It improves the quality of life.

The lifestyle recommended in the book is not only for the obese population, but for everyone. Every person should accept it for the promotion of health. Certain environmental factors like pollution, global warming, uncontrolled population, computer exposure, stress and competition are unavoidable circumstances in modern society. We are progressing fast and the side effects of progress are affecting our health. To enjoy the fruits of progress, we have to preserve, promote and progress our health up to the optimum level. We have to bequeath good health to our next generation. We have to build a strong, fit and progressing world. Accept a **healthy lifestyle** and be strong and healthy.

Chapter 19

Obesity and Cardiovascular Diseases

Dr. Jagdish Hiremath
D.M. DNB

Dr. Sanika Mijar
B.H.M.S. PPHC

There is mounting evidence relating obesity to cardiovascular diseases (CVD). With technological advances, jobs have become more sedentary and production of large quantities of cheap food has increased. These lead to an increasing number of future cardiovascular events, which are attributable to obesity. Even more alarming are reports that show increasing obesity rates in children and young people. The effects on cardiovascular events will be more evident when the young obese approach middle age. It is widely known that obesity leads to the development of hypertension, diabetes mellitus, sleep apnea, hyperlipidemia (high cholesterol) and all classic contributors of CVD.

Research, over the past decade, has shown that obesity promotes a state of inflammation in parallel; coronary heart disease (CHD) has been recognized as resulting from inflammatory processes in atheromatous plaques. Obesity also causes insulin resistance (ineffective insulin) and elevated insulin levels that are linked to atherosclerosis. There is an increasing weightage to the role of intra-abdominal fat, estimated by the waist circumference, which is associated with insulin resistance syndrome, sleep apnea and inflammation—three potentially critical players in the obesity-CVD link.

Effects of Obesity on Cardiac Structure and Function

Obesity is characterized by the addition of fat mass as well as muscles, organs (viscera) and skin, all of which increase oxygen consumption. The heart has to work hard to supply blood to every nook and corner of an obese person's body. Thickened arteries and veins make this task still more difficult. The total blood volume and plasma volume increase in proportion to the degree of obesity. This leads to cardio megaly (enlarged heart). The initial response to increased metabolic demand and total blood volume is chamber dilation, which over time leads to increased mass of the heart. This leads to increased radius and wall thickness of heart chambers. Hypertension, which is common in obesity, exaggerates this enlargement.

Association of Obesity with Cardiovascular Morbidity and Mortality

Generalized obesity

The relationship between obesity and death is clearly evident. Increasing obesity has a direct relationship with increase in heart related deaths. In addition, obesity has been associated with enlarged heart and hypertension with a high rate of heart failure.

Visceral Obesity (Fat Deposition in Organs): A Better Predictor

Central or abdominal obesity is associated with insulin resistance, high blood pressure and exaggerated cholesterol levels. Blood viscosity is also elevated in central obesity in comparison with generalized obesity and may contribute to a greater coronary risk. Waist circumference is a fair reflection of abdominal fat and is easy to measure. It must be remembered that waist circumference measures the magnitude of both visceral fat and fat under the skin around the belly alone. Waist circumference greater than 80 cm in women or 90 cm in men has been shown to be associated with increased risk of CVD in India. Waist circumference above these thresholds indicates need for intervention even if the patient does not fall in the obese category. Visceral fat deposition generally is greater in men than in women and increases with aging and after menopause in women.

Epidemiology of Cardiovascular Disease in Obesity

Low Birth Weight

Low birth weight babies generally grow obese in childhood and adulthood due overfeeding. They show a higher risk to CVD.

Obesity and Blood Pressure

Hypertension is defined as a systolic blood pressure ≥ 140mm Hg or a diastolic blood pressure ≥ 90mm. Hg is one of the most important preventable causes for premature deaths worldwide, contributing to approximately half of all CVD worldwide. In many countries, up to 30% of adults have hypertension; about 50–60% would be in better health in future if they reduce their blood pressure by increasing physical activity, maintaining an ideal body weight and eating more fruits and vegetables. CVD doubles for every 10-mm Hg increase in diastolic blood pressure or every 20 mm-Hg increase in systolic blood pressure. The link between obesity and hypertension has been largely explained. For each 1 kg/m^2 increment in current BMI, the risk of hypertension increases by 12%. Women with BMI above 31 have a risk compared with the leanest women. Weight gain of 1 kg after age 18 years elevates the risk of hypertension by 5%.

Lifestyle recommendations for blood pressure control:

- Weight reduction in overweight individuals

- Reduction of salt intake to < 6 g daily (one tablespoon full)

- Avoidance and restriction of alcohol consumption

- Regular physical activity in sedentary individuals

- Quitting smoking

- Dietary changes

Obesity and Dyslipidemia (High Cholesterol and Other Fats)

Obesity and insulin resistance both strongly affect fat metabolism and classically lead to higher low-density lipoprotein cholesterol (LDLC), TG and lower HDLC. Weight loss reduces TG (triglycerides) and LDLC and increases HDLC. Rates of cholesterol production correlate with excess body fat, with an approximately 20 mg/dl increase per kg rise in body fat. As with other coronary risk factors, visceral fat may impact many of these relationships. Weight reduction through caloric restriction has been associated with significant reductions in LDLC. The effects of diet and weight loss on changes in HDLC have been more variable. However, weight loss occurs with prolonged low saturated fat diet but HDLC returns to the baseline. The increase in HDLC produced by dietary restriction alone is consistently less for women than for men. For men, aerobic exercise and diet increase HDLC significantly more than diet alone.

Obstructive Sleep Apnea (OSA)

In a large population in which sleep studies were performed, obesity was a major risk factor for the prevalence of sleep disorder and breathing problem. Cardiovascular risk is worsened by many of the effects of obesity, wherein OSA acts a mediator. Interestingly, OSA patients have a greater proportion of visceral fat than obese people without sleep apnea. OSA is a significant prediction of both systolic and diastolic blood pressures, independent of age, BMI and sex. Each additional apnea per hour increases the chance of hypertension by 1%. OSA leads to a markedly increased pressure in the arteries of the lung (PAH). The most successful therapy for OSA is bariatric surgery. Weight loss through diet was shown to be associated with decrease in upper airway collapsibility in OSA.

Endothelial Dysfunction

Endothelium is the inner smooth lining of arteries and is the most important 'organ' of the body. Roughening of the endothelium and its malfunction lead to dysfunction of various organs and finally leads to atherosclerosis and blockages in the arteries. Endothelial dysfunction is considered the earliest manifestation of atherosclerosis. A normal endothelium has the ability to expand and allow more flow in the organs under stress or with exercise. It can lose this ability later. Then a chain of events over a period of years leads to atherosclerosis. Obesity directly correlates with endothelial dysfunction. High insulin levels, insulin resistance, high glucoses levels, high blood pressure and many other associations of obesity cause endothelial dysfunction. Fortunately, it is reversible to a large extent with weight reduction.

Problems Associated with Treatment of Obese Cardiac Patients

- High-risk individuals with multiple risk factors
- Higher doses required according to weight
- Higher complication rates
- Longer time taken and problems related to anesthesia during surgery
- Post-operative complications like prolonged ventilation, low oxygenation, poor breathing efforts and deep vein thrombosis
- Prolonged recovery, poor rehabilitation

Aims for Primary Prevention of CVD

BMI   :   Within 10% of normal

BP   :   < 140/90 mm of Hg

TG   :   < 200 mg%

LDL   :   < 100 mg%

HDL   :   > 40 mg%

Sugars   :   < 150 mg%

Aims for Secondary Prevention of CVD

(Diabetic or any other vascular disease)

BMI   :   Within 10% normal

BP   :   < 120/80 mm of Hg

TG   :   < 150 mg%

LDL   :   < 70 mg%

HDL   :   < 45 mg%

Sugars   :   < 150 mg%

Prevention and Reversal of CVD

Dr. Sumedha Bhosale

The information above indicates, in a clear-cut way, that the contributory factors or risk factors to coronary heart diseases are preventable and reversible. If you practice a healthy lifestyle, approximately 90% of risk factors for CVD can be prevented.

Let us see the leading risk factors to the development of CVD.

- Physical inactivity

- High blood pressure

- Excessive body fat

- Low HDL (good) cholesterol

- Elevated LDL (bad) cholesterol

- Elevated triglycerides

- Elevated homocysteine

- Diabetes

- Abnormal ECG

- Tobacco

- Stress

- Personal and family history of CVD

- Age

- Gender

Physical Inactivity

Improving cardio-respiratory endurance through aerobic exercise has perhaps the greatest impact in reducing the overall risk of CVD. In the present scenario of modern mechanized societies, we cannot afford not to exercise. Research shows that aerobic exercise is extremely beneficial in reducing cardiovascular diseases.

Moderate amount of aerobic exercise can reduce cardiovascular risk considerably. A regular aerobic exercise program helps control most of the major risk factors that lead to heart and blood vessel diseases.

Aerobic exercise will:

- increase cardio-respiratory endurance.

- decrease and control blood pressure.

- reduce body fat.

- lower blood lipids (cholesterol and triglycerides).

- improve HDL cholesterol (refer to next page).

- help control or decrease the risk of diabetes. (Refer to chapter __, page __.)

- increase and maintain good heart function, sometimes improving certain ECG abnormalities.

- motivate toward smoking cessation.

- alleviate stress.

- counteract the personal history of heart disease.

Hypertension

Hypertension, when it is mild or borderline, can be controlled without medication but with changes in lifestyle such as regular aerobic exercise, weight control, a low-salt, low-fat and high-potassium/high-calcium diet, lowered alcohol and caffeine intake, smoking cessation and stress management. If blood pressure is significantly above normal, then medication is necessary.

Aerobic exercise gives individuals an induced reduction of approximately 4.5 mm Hg in resting systolic blood pressure and 3–4 mm Hg in resting diastolic blood pressure. You may feel that these reductions are not huge, but remember that even a 5-mm Hg decrease in diastolic pressure has been associated with 40% decrease in risk of stroke and 15% decrease in coronary heart disease. A hypertensive person who exercises has a lower risk of mortality.

Exercise is more important than weight reduction

(Weight reduction without exercise will not be helpful to control hypertension.)

The effects of at least four weeks of strength training in gym also yield similar results.

A few things are worth noting during the exercise.

- Check pre- and post-exercise blood pressure to modify the intensity of exercise.

- Use minimum resistance (weights) in terms of dumbbells, machines or barbells and perform maximum repetition.

- Do not hold the breath, as this may lead to sudden rise in BP and may lead to complications like stroke.

- If you feel any abnormal symptoms, then immediately stop the exercise and inform the physician about it.

- Before starting your exercise, always discuss with your consultant, instructor, dietician and physician the type, mode, frequency and intensity of the exercise.

A healthy lifestyle is extremely useful and extremely necessary to control and maintain the blood pressure.

Obesity

Obesity is recognized as a major risk factor for CVD along with other chronic disorders.

Maintaining recommended body weight (fat percentage) is essential in any cardiovascular risk reduction program. Even a modest weight reduction of 5–10% can reduce high blood pressure and cholesterol level.

Healthy lifestyle is the treatment for obesity.

Abnormal cholesterol profile: Triglycerides, total cholesterol, high-density lipoproteins and low-density lipoproteins are considered in the blood lipid test. A poor blood lipid profile is thought to be the most important predisposing factor in the development of CVD. The general recommendation is to keep total cholesterol below 200 mg/dl, LDL cholesterol below 130 mg/dl, triglycerides below 125 mg/dl and HDL above 45 mg/dl.

HDL acts as 'scavengers,' removing cholesterol from the body and preventing plaque formation. The protein molecules found in the coating of HDL come in contact with cholesterol-filled cells, get attached to the cells and take their cholesterol.

LDL tends to release the cholesterol, which may then penetrate the linings of arteries and speed up the process of atherosclerosis. Genetically found, LP (a) is a variation of LDL responsible for atherosclerosis. HDL, the good cholesterol, offers some protection against CVD. Habitual aerobic exercise, gym exercise, weight loss, niacin and quitting smoking help raise HDL. Beta carotene may also promote higher HDL cholesterol level. More the intensity of aerobic exercise, higher the level of HDL.

LDL cholesterol, which is bad cholesterol, comes in contact with free radicals and get oxidized. At this time, white blood cells invade the arterial wall, take up the cholesterol and clog the arteries. The anti-radicals or antioxidants, vitamin C and E, beta carotene and selenium can reduce the risk of CVD.

A single unstable free radical can damage or oxidize LDL particles. Vitamin C inactivates free radicals, vitamin E protects LDL from oxidation, and beta carotene absorbs free radicals and keeps them from causing damage. Beta carotene may also help cause an increase in HDL levels. One or two medium-sized raw carrots per day provide the recommended daily amount of beta carotene antioxidant nutrients.

Saturated fats raise cholesterol levels more than anything else in the diet. Red meat and dairy products are the sources rich in saturated fats. It is better to avoid them. Unsaturated fats cannot be converted into cholesterol.

Lowering LDL Cholesterol

If LDL cholesterol is higher, then it can be lowered by losing body fat, by consuming low-cal, nutritious and balanced diet and also by participating in a regular aerobic exercise program.

Even though medication helps lower LDL cholesterol, it is better to lower it without it and practice a healthy lifestyle, because drugs used to lower the cholesterol can cause muscle and joint pain and can alter the liver enzyme level. In the presence of heart disease, even if medication is prescribed, we must combine it with a healthy lifestyle.

To decrease LDL cholesterol, the diet should be low in fat, low in cholesterol, high in fiber and without saturated fats. Use of poly unsaturated and mono unsaturated fats, instead of saturated fats, tends to decrease LDL cholesterol.

Exercise is important, as dietary modifications alone are as not as effective as a combination of diet plus aerobic exercise.

Triglycerides are also known as free fatty acids. In combination with cholesterol, they speed up the formation of plaque. They are found in red meat, skin, shell fish, honey, alcohol and free sugars. They significantly raise triglycerides levels. Weight reduction with reduction in such foods helps bring down the triglyceride level below 100 mg/dl.

Elevated Homocysteine

Homocysteine is used by the body to help build proteins and carry out cellular metabolism. During an intermediate step, homocysteine leads to creation of another amino acid. This process requires the presence of folate, vitamin 86 and B12. Homocysteine accumulation is toxic, because it may:

- damage the inner lining of arteries (the initial step in the process of atherosclerosis).

- stimulate the proliferation of cells that contribute to plaque formation.

- encourage clotting that may completely obstruct the blood flow in an artery.

Five servings of vegetables, fruits, grains, meat and legume every day give folate and 86 required in removing and clearing homocysteine from the blood. An additional supplement of B complex is not necessary, if you have five servings of vegetables and fruits daily. Vitamin 812 found in 1 cup milk or 1 egg fulfills the daily requirement.

Diabetes: Refer to Chapter 18

Cigarette Smoking

It is closely associated with CVD (like cancer, peptic ulcers, bronchitis and emphysema). Passive smoking is equally risky for adults and children.

Smoking speeds up the process of atherosclerosis and also increases risk of sudden death by three times following myocardial infarction (heart attack). Smoking increases heart rate and blood pressure and irritates the heart, which can trigger fatal arrhythmias (irregular heart rhythm).

Another harmful effect is decrease in HDL cholesterol, the 'good' cholesterol that helps control blood lipid profile.

The moment a person quits the smoking, the risk for CVD starts to decrease. Chewing tobacco and smoking pipe and cigar are equally bad. Even though you do not inhale smoke, toxic substances are absorbed through the membrane and enter the blood stream. Exercise and weight loss help in quitting smoking stress.

Stress

Due to stress, more catecholamines (brain hormone) are secreted to prepare the body for fight or flight. If stress is not relieved, they remain elevated in the blood stream. This leads to constriction of coronary arteries, leading to reduced oxygen supply to the heart. If blood vessels are largely blocked, due to atherosclerosis, then abnormal heart rhythm or even a heart attack may follow.

Physical activity is one of the best ways to relieve stress. Physical activity leads to metabolism of excess catecholamine and brings it to the normal level.

Muscular activity causes muscular relaxation. Exercise burns up excess tension along with excess calories. Exercise causes secretion of happy hormones like endorphin, which gives a calming effect. It is the best mode of relaxation.

Personal and Family History

If there is a history of CVD in your family or if you have a personal history of CVD, then the best way to keep them away is to commit to a healthy lifestyle, which is the only way to decrease the future risk significantly.

Age and Gender

Women above 55 and men above 45 are found to have more risk of CVD. It seems as we grow older, we tend to be less physically active, less caring about nutrition, and tend to get obese. These factors may be the reasons for increased risk of CVD at this age along with aging.

Young people should not think that they are safe. The process begins early in life. Elevated cholesterol levels at the age of 10, atherosclerosis at the age of 12, and maturity onset diabetes at the age of 8 are the findings from latest studies in the last two years.

It is true that the aging process cannot be stopped. But it certainly can be slowed down. In longevity, the concept of chronological age versus physiological age is important. Some individuals above the age of 60 have the fitness of 35 years old and vice versa. Accepting a healthy lifestyle is the only way to slow down natural aging.

Chapter 20

Obesity and Polycystic Ovarian Syndrome (PCOS)

Dr. Sanjay Gupte
M.D., D.G.O., F.I.C.O.G

Polycystic ovarian syndrome is a health condition linked to hormone imbalance and insulin resistance. About 10% of women suffer from PCOS. This disorder of PCOS is brought forward by certain symptoms, which are as follows:

Irregular Menstrual Periods

This is marked by menstrual cycles of fewer than 21 days, greater than 35 days, and more than 4 days variation. Sometimes, it causes the absence of menstrual period i.e. amenorrhea. Consistently irregular menstrual periods with long gaps causes oligomenorrhoea acne, pimples on the face but sometimes on the shoulder back and chest too.

Fatigue and depression are other symptoms.

Hair related issues: Male type hair loss, i.e. thinning of the hair from the crown on the head, is common. Excess body hair and facial hair is known as hirsutism. It has a pattern of distribution that is common among males. These symptoms may be mild or severe and can vary widely from one woman to other. Many times, the symptoms of this syndrome can be misdiagnosed as stress or premenstrual syndrome.

In women with this syndrome, the ovaries are not capable of producing the correct balance of female hormones. Because of this imbalance, the ovaries cannot develop the ovum i.e. eggs or they cannot release them. This leads to the formation of empty egg follicles on the ovary. This empty egg follicle is known as cyst. Polycystic ovaries mean ovaries with many cysts. Polycystic ovaries have a string of these empty follicles around their outside. There are usually 10 or more cysts. The size of the cyst varies from 2 mm to 8 mm. The tissue within the ovary gets thickened and is called as stroma. When 10 cysts with a thickened stroma are present, then it enables the diagnosis of the condition of polycystic ovaries. This diagnosis is done by using ultrasound scan to view the ovaries.

PCOS is not ovarian cyst. Ovarian cysts are usually single and can grow bigger. Ovarian cyst interferes with ovarian function. Polycystic ovarian cysts are different than ovarian cysts. In PCOS, the string of tiny cysts, which are empty egg follicles that have failed to develop completely and release an egg, appears outside the ovary. PCO cysts are symptoms. They are due to a deep underlying hormonal and metabolic problem.

The treatment of this cyst is not surgical removal. In fact, you have to sort out the underlying problems thorough change in diet, exercise and medication, if needed. Here we treat the cause of PCOS to get rid of the other symptoms, along with PCO cysts. With this treatment, the cysts can be reduced in number.

The Causes of PCOS

In 1935, it was thought for the first time that PCOS was a condition due to hormonal imbalance. Elevated levels of luteinizing hormone (LH female hormone) have been found in some woman but not all have PCOS. Elevated levels of testosterone hormone (TH male hormone) are also associated with PCOS and its symptoms. Testosterone inhibits ovulation and causes menstrual irregularities. Inappropriate levels of LH and testosterone are again symptoms due to other disorders and cannot be the cause of PCOS.

Recent research is focused on elevated insulin levels in some women with PCOS. Elevated levels of insulin in women with PCOS promote androgen (male hormone) production by the ovaries. This contributes to the disturbances in menstruation. But all women do not have elevated insulin levels, even though they have PCOS. It is not a single cause of problem. PCOS is a complex disorder generated by a number of factors. It is well known that PCOS seems to run in families. The genes controlling androgen and insulin production may play the main role in PCOS. However, other genetic factors may affect the type and severity of the symptoms. In addition, environmental issues such as lifestyle, diet, obesity and pollution play an important role in the development and control of the symptoms.

- **Symptoms:** Obesity or being overweight, irregular or absent periods, infertility and overgrowth of facial or body hair are thought to be classic symptoms. Additionally, fatigue, joint pain, hair loss (alopecia,) tenderness in breasts, bloating, diabetes with insulin resistance, mood swings and depression are the symptoms presented and reported by patients associated with PCOS. Other symptoms include pelvic pain, breast pain, abdominal pain, dizziness and increased tendency to faint. A woman with PCOS can have any single or combination of any or all these symptoms. Generally, the symptoms tend to get worse over time, with weight gain, and lead to obesity.

Even if the periods are consistently irregular or absent, the chances are that ovulation is irregular or it does not occur at all. This leads to delay in conceiving. Being diagnosed with PCOS does not mean that you are infertile. Many women conceive without any problems. Some women find it a little harder to get pregnant but they manage without medical intervention. Other women need fertility treatment, either drug-based or just by using nutritional and natural therapies. Women with PCOS can have problems in losing weight.

The PCOS Weight Trap

In women with PCOS, it is found that TEF (thermic effect of food; refer to page _) is reduced. This leads to weight gain. It is also thought that higher than average levels of testosterone (which all women with PCOS have) are linked with a tendency to hold fats.

Added to this is the insulin-resistance-problem, which blocks the action of hormones that can help in burning fat and energy and also sets a trap of a cycle of ups and downs in blood sugar, leading to trapping the person in a PCOS weight trap. The patient craves foods that give the blood a sugar rush. The sugar is stored and the person puts on weight without being able to shift it anywhere. In other words, a woman with PCOS who eats the same seven days' worth of food may store calories equal to eight days' worth. Obesity is a frequent feature of PCOS although its presence is not required for diagnosis. At least 50% of women with PCOS are obese. Excess body weight can influence both the metabolic and reproductive features of PCOS. Obesity also has significant implications for the response to treatment for infertility, menstrual dysfunction and metabolic abnormalities. Obesity may also influence pregnancy outcomes in PCOS.

During adolescence, girls start gaining weight and become obese. In the last two decades, the rate of obesity has become three times than before. Obesity has an adverse impact on reproductive as well as metabolic features of PCOS. It is advocated that everyone should change their lifestyle by accepting the healthy lifestyle practices described in this book to lose and maintain the weight at a normal value.

Impact on Reproductive Process

Menstrual Dysfunction and Infertility

Menstrual dysfunction is one of the defining features of PCOS. Even though women with PCOS have regular menstrual cycles, they are not consistently ovulatory. Obesity is associated with menstrual disturbances and an increased frequency of an ovulatory cycles. Endometrium, the inner most layer of the uterus, is exposed to estrogen at a high level. This increased exposure is unopposed by the progesterone. This leads to increased risk of hyperplasia and cancer of the endometrium. About 40% of endometrial cancers are related to obesity. Women with BMI > 29 kg/sq.m. have a three-fold greater risk of endometrial cancer.

In obesity, the risk of infertility is also increased. Obesity leads to ovulatory dysfunction. Obese women require more ovulatory induction agents. Women with BMI > 24 to 32, have a 1.3-fold higher risk of infertility; with BMI > 32 they have a 2.7-fold higher risk of infertility.

Endocrine Impact of Obesity

Hyper-androgenism or PCOS is positively correlated with the degree of insulin resistance, independent of obesity. Obesity in PCOS, however, is associated with more severe insulin resistance compared to lean women with PCOS.

Metabolic Disturbance and Obesity in PCOS

Obesity impacts the reproductive and endocrine features of PCOS. It also impacts metabolic features more dramatically. Women with PCOS are insulin-resistant. This contributes to significant metabolic abnormalities that are seen in PCOS.

Insulin resistance is strongly influenced by the presence of obesity. Thus, there is synergetic contribution of obesity to insulin resistance in PCOS. In fact, the contribution of obesity to the manifestation of insulin resistance, resulting in metabolic disorder, is more important than that of PCOS itself. One of the most dramatic findings of the influence of PCOS in metabolic disease is the impact on glucose tolerance. Glucose intolerance in PCOS has increased at a faster rate in the general population. This rate is also significantly influenced by the presence of obesity.

Cardiovascular Risk in PCOS

There is an association of increased cardiovascular risk factors with PCOS. These risk factors are increased by obesity. Obese women with PCOS are at a potentially higher risk for CVD. Women with PCOS have higher total cholesterol and triglycerides. Additionally, these women have increased arterial stiffness and decreased flow-mediated vasodilatation.

Weight Loss and PCOS

Weight reduction with a healthy lifestyle shows an improvement in reproductive parameters. The menstruation cyclicity improves. A low-cal balanced diet significantly improves both menstrual cyclicity and ovulation. A low-cal balanced diet along with exercise may cause return of spontaneous ovulation and the chances of becoming naturally pregnant, in many cases. Weight reduction is always recommended as a primary therapy before use of ovulation-induction agents for fertility, according to some experts.

Women with PCOS, who desire to conceive, should set the goal of achieving normal body weight. A clearly modest weight loss may improve ovulatory function. Such patients must be educated about the impact of obesity on the potential of fertility and on the complications of pregnancy.

Weight reduction through a healthy lifestyle is fundamental in the treatment of such individuals. Scientific exercise, balanced nutritious diet, good relaxation techniques and good rest are very important during weight reduction.

Weight Loss and Endometrial Cancer

We have read earlier in this chapter that sustained unopposed estrogen in a chronic an ovulatory state leads to a greater risk of cancer of endometrium in obese women with PCOS.

Women who have sustained some degree of weight loss have a lower risk for endometrial cancer. If you can sustain weight loss for 5 years or more, you can derive 25% lower risk of developing endometrial cancer.

Lifestyle Management in Adolescents

If weight reduction through a healthy lifestyle is achieved in adolescence, it could have a significant positive impact on the reproductive course of the disease. After weight reduction in adolescence, many times there is androgen reduction in hypo-androgenism and PCOS.

In obese adolescent girls, even an average reduction of 9% of body weight, with a healthy lifestyle, leads to reduction in testosterone. If you not do reduce weight at this stage, then there is a further weight gain and increase in testosterone. Androgen is sensitive to weight reduction in obese adolescent girls.

Summary

- There is substantial evidence that obesity is associated with reproduction and metabolic complications in PCOS.

- Significant increase in insulin resistance associated with obesity has implications of disease well past the reproductive years.

- A healthy lifestyle with scientific exercise, balanced, nutritious low-cal diet, rest and relaxation, and positive mental attitude (prescribed in this book) is a well-established treatment for metabolic disease and prevention and management of type II diabetes mellitus.

- These interventions are extremely successful in improving the reproductive process and presumably similar metabolic improvements over time.

- Weight reduction in PCOS shows considerable increase in the conception rate.

- Weight reduction in adolescence is helpful in controlling testosterone values, according to some studies

Things to Remember during Weight Reduction Program with PCOS

Dr. Sumedha Bhosale

Due to amenorrhea and hormonal disturbances, many times, in spite of perfect treatment of exercise and calorie control, there may not be any visible change in weight, during some specific period due to water retention.

The same symptoms are experienced as described in premenstrual syndrome (page _). You have to continue with your everyday routine planned by your consultant. Water retention is responsible in this situation for weight gain or not reduction in weight.

Drink lots of water and if possible drink plain coconut water. This will help reduce water retention, as water consumption in enough quantity works as a diuretic and reduces retention. Do not worry as controlling calories and expending them through exercise always creates a negative energy balance, which causes reduction in fat percentage and measurements.

Exercise improves the metabolism of hormones. TEE, TEF, obligatory and adaptive thermic effects help raise the BMR. Reduction in fat percentage improves the insulin action. Even though your weight reduction is comparatively at a slower rate in the beginning, slowly and steadily you can achieve the goal of weight reduction.

Do not get disturbed. Think positively. If you are taking treatment for conception, then it is advisable to lose your extra weight prior to medication. Many women conceive naturally without medication when they lose some extra weight. Other women with the same problems may expect the same results with weight reduction. Every woman is different. Some may need medication, others may require a longer period to reduce weight. Remember that there are so many factors responsible for infertility. Do not get disappointed during every menstruation cycle, after starting treatment of weight reduction. Always feel proud about your achievements.

- If your menstruation cycle is painful, you can try light exercise with some stretches. Do not think about calorie expenditure during menstruation. Light exercises help you relieve pain. Do not forget to follow a proper diet meticulously during this period.

- If periods are normal and without pain, you can do the exercises like the other days.

- Keep yourself busy in some creative work. Do not keep thinking about the same issue continuously.

- For weight reduction in adolescents, read the chapter on prevention of obesity.

- Even after conception, stick to a healthy lifestyle after consultation with your gynecologist.

- In some cases, bed rest during pregnancy is advised. So, take care to take the advice of your gynecologist prior to continuing your exercise and consumption of a low-sugar diet. You must not restart junk and high-cal deep-fried food.

Chapter 21

Obesity and Pregnancy

Dr. Parag Biniwale
M.D. (Obgyn.) F.I.C.O.G.,
F.I.C.M.C.H.,
Diploma in pelviscopic surgery (Germany)

A healthy pregnancy is one without physical or psychological pathology in the mother or the fetus and results in the delivery of a healthy baby. There was a time when obesity was thought to be a problem of Western countries. Now, pregnant women in India too are becoming overweight and obese, adding a lot of problems to the growing fetus and themselves. It's more difficult for women to get pregnant when they are overweight. Even if they conceive, the risk of complications during pregnancy and the problems for the baby after birth increase dramatically.

Weight gain in pregnancy averages to 11–13 kg but it varies depending on the mother's pre-pregnancy weight. A very thin woman who is below her optimum weight should gain 14–16 kg, while an overweight or obese woman should gain 6–7 kg. The most crucial factor is the pattern of weight gain during pregnancy. In one study, excess weight gain early in pregnancy was a strong predictor of how much weight the women retained after delivery. A steady but gradual weight gain is recommended during the first two trimesters with the bulk of the weight gained during the last trimester, the period when the baby is adding weight and growing at the fastest rate.

Nowadays, girls start putting on weight in adolescence itself. Hence, the weight gained during pregnancy is always greater when compared to the weight gained during pregnancy 25 years ago.

Problems in Pregnancy Due to Obesity

All pregnant women have a risk of pregnancy complications. However, most pregnancies are uncomplicated. Obesity increases the risk of a number of pregnancy complications. The more obese you are, the more your level of risk rises. Overweight or obese women are at an increased risk of having complications during pregnancy. These complications include gestational diabetes, pre-eclampsia (a disorder that occurs only during pregnancy with high blood pressure, swelling of feet and protein in urine; this affects both the mother and the unborn baby) or eclampsia (high blood pressure, protein in urine, fits) and hospitalization.

The risk of the mother being hospitalized during pregnancy goes up 4 times if she's overweight. If her BMI is over 35, the risk goes up 6–7 times. The risk of prenatal mortality also increases as maternal BMI increases.

Overweight women are at an increased risk of the following pregnancy complications:

Before Pregnancy

- Obese women require a longer time to become pregnant than others. The average time taken by obese women to become pregnant is significantly longer (11 months) than women with normal weight and overweight women (7–8 months).

- Many obese women have polycystic ovarian syndrome with irregular menses, which can interfere with ovulation. (Refer to chapter _ by Dr. Sanjay Gupte.)

During Pregnancy

- Women who are obese during pregnancy are more likely to have gestational diabetes and problems with labor and delivery.

- Pre-eclampsia is a condition that occurs only in pregnancy, characterized by hypertension (high blood pressure) and presence of protein in the urine. Obesity during pregnancy is associated with increased risk of death for both the baby and the mother and increases the risk of maternal high blood pressure by 10 times. Pre-eclampsia, which can lead to seizures, premature delivery, fetal distress and death, is seen more frequently in obese women.

- Abnormalities in the baby's growth, development and general health obesity during pregnancy is associated with increased risk of birth defects, particularly neural tube defects, such as spina bifida. There are reports that show that women who are overweight or obese are 30–40% more likely to deliver a baby with a major birth defect, such as one that affects the brain, heart, and digestive system.

- Sleep apnea is a condition that causes you to temporarily stop breathing while you are sleeping.

- Prenatal care is complicated because measurements of uterine size and ultrasound tests can be more difficult. This can make accurate prediction of your due date a bit of a problem.

During Labor

- Failure to progress in labor

- Shoulder dystocia (the shoulders of the baby gets stuck during birth)

- Difficulties while monitoring the baby's heart beats

- Difficulty in providing satisfactory pain relief in labor

- Increased risks with attempted vaginal birth after Cesarean section

- Need for an emergency Cesarean section

- Increased risk of complications related to Cesarean section

- Infants born to women who are obese during pregnancy are more likely to have high birth weight and low blood sugar (which can be associated with brain damage and seizures).

After Child Birth

- Increased risk of wound infection

- Increased risk of blood clots (particularly following a Cesarean section)

- Post-natal depression

Obesity and Cesarean Section

The problems of operating on women with obesity

- Positioning is difficult because women are unable to lie flat and have to be moved if an emergency arises.

- An epidural or spinal anesthesia is more difficult to site correctly and is more likely to dislodge or fail.

- It is more difficult to maintain airways (especially in the emergency setting).

- Surgical procedure is more difficult.

- Extra monitoring is required.

- The patient may require admission to an intensive care unit after the operation.

- Complications of Cesarean delivery, such as wound infection and life-threatening pulmonary embolus (a blockage of an artery in the lungs by fat, air, tumor tissue, or blood clot), are also more likely

- Despite these problems, obese women are more likely to require a Cesarean section for a wide range of conditions/problems. Considering all issues related to the patient and baby, the doctor may recommend an elective Cesarean section.

Diet and Exercise Tips for Two

There is a common disbelief that a pregnant woman should eat for two people. However, we must remember that her calorie requirement increases only by 300 calories and not by 2,200 calories.

To achieve a small but steady weight gain, the overweight women needs to focus on a nutrient-dense diet. Foods that are nutrient-dense provide a high nutrientto-calorie ratio. For e.g., whole grains, beans and legumes, vegetables, fruits, low-fat dairy products, and lean protein sources. Foods with low nutrient density contribute fat and/or sugar to the diet along with a few other nutrients.

The daily diet should consist of 9–11 servings of grains (emphasizing whole grains), 3–4 servings of vegetables, 3–4 servings of fruits, 4 servings of low-fat dairy products or calcium-fortified soy products and 6 or more ounces of a protein source. Eating small and frequent meals and snacks made up of nutritious foods is the best way to increase calorie intake. While exercise is an important component of a healthy pregnancy, it is vital that her physician or health counselor evaluates the overweight pregnant woman before starting an exercise program.

Refer to the chapter below by Dr. Sumedha Bhosale.

As the extra weight puts more demands on the body, it's especially important to warm up, cool down and follow exercise guidelines for pregnant women. Above all, a pregnant woman should listen to her own body. If she feels discomfort, she should stop immediately.

Low-intensity activities, such as walking, swimming and low-impact exercises classes designed for the pregnant woman, can contribute to better health for both mother and baby. Due to the risk of gestational diabetes, it is important for women to avoid dehydration by drinking plenty of fluids while exercising and not become overheated during physical activity. Besides, women can ensure a healthy pregnancy and baby by being in shape before pregnancy. Weight loss is not recommended during pregnancy.

Weight matters: For the health of both mother and baby, women of childbearing age and their health consultant should work together to assess and address this important health issue before, during and after pregnancy. The health counselor can do the following:

Recommendations for all women (including women in the pre-conception period)

- Inform and counsel women about the health risks associated with overweight and obesity.

- Encourage a healthy diet.

- Screen for hypertension and diabetes mellitus in women who are at risk.

- Counsel women to consume adequate folic acid, iron and calcium.

- Encourage regular exercise (>30 minutes of moderate physical activity daily).

- Counsel women to quit smoking.

- Counsel women to avoid consuming alcohol during pregnancy.

Recommendations during pregnancy (prenatal) for all/women

- Encourage a healthy diet.

- Discuss recommended weight gain during pregnancy.

Recommendations after pregnancy (postnatal) for all women

- Encourage breastfeeding.

- Counsel women to return to a healthy weight.

Pregnancy and Exercise

Dr. Sumedha Bhosale

Women should not avoid exercise during pregnancy. They should exercise to strengthen the body and prepare for delivery. Moderate exercise during pregnancy helps prevent excessive weight gain and speeds up the recovery following the delivery.

Pregnant women in the lower socio-economic class do difficult work up to the very last day of delivery. A few hours after the baby's birth, they resume their normal activities. Women athletes have competed in sports during early stages of pregnancy. The pregnant woman, her physician, gynecologist and health consultant should make the final decision regarding the exercise program.

Word of Caution

Stretching exercises are to be performed gently because hormonal changes during pregnancy increase laxity of muscles and connective tissues to facilitate delivery. They make women more susceptible to injuries during exercise.

Guidelines for Exercise during Pregnancy

For pregnant women without any risk and who have the approval of the gynecologist and physician:

- Continue to exercise at a mild-to-moderate pace throughout the pregnancy but decrease the exercise intensity by about 25% from the pre-pregnancy program.

- Exercise regularly for a minimum of three times a week instead of the occasional exercise bouts.

- Pay attention to the body's signals of discomfort and distress. Stop the exercise when tired. Never exercise to exhaustion. Stop if unusual symptoms arise, such as pain of any kind, cramping, nausea, bleeding, leaking of amniotic fluid, faintness, dizziness, palpitations, numbness in any part of the body, or decreased fetal activity.

- After the first trimester, avoid exercises that require you to lie on your back. This position can block the blood flow to the uterus and the baby.

- Do non-weight-bearing activities such as cycling, swimming, or water aerobics, which minimize the risk of injury and allow continuation of exercise throughout pregnancy.

- Avoid activities that could precipitate a loss of balance or cause even mild trauma to the abdomen.

- Get proper nourishment. (Pregnancy requires approximately 300 extra calories per day.) During the first three months in particular, avoid exercising in the heat. Wear clothing that allows proper dissipation of heat, and drink plenty of water.

Chapter 22

Obesity and Menopause

Dr. Vaishali Parag Biniwale
M.D., D.G.O

Menopause can be described as a change in life. In other words, the menstruation cycle stops during this period, which may last from a few months to a few years. The average age of menopause is between 45 to 53 ± 5 years. If you do not have menstrual period flow for 12 months, then you are said to have entered the post-menopausal phase.

Menopause is the result of decreased estrogen (female hormone) production by the ovaries. Estrogen hormone is extremely useful in the health aspect of every woman. It has been reported that estrogen has protective effects in 72 probable diseases of women. The important benefits of estrogen are on skin, hair, breasts, uterus, other external reproductive organs, urinary system, bones and blood vessels. We discussed earlier that the metabolism of fats is affected negatively by lack of estrogen, which affects fat distribution and body composition.

The menopausal symptoms in totality are known as 'menopause syndrome.' Menopausal women are deprived of the protective effects of estrogen. Psychological changes such as insomnia (sleeplessness), irritation, depression, lack of concentration, fatigue, inability to take decision and lack of interest in sex are significant. These negative psychological changes, along with lack of physical activity and deprivation of the benefits of estrogen, synergistically tend to lead to obesity in women during the peri-menopausal period.

Obesity, adverse changes in fat distribution and body composition, increased risk of coronary heart disease and heart attack, increased cholesterol, high blood pressure, insulin resistance are some of the significant adverse conditions due to menopause, characterized by lack of estrogen as well as increased weight. About 20% of menopausal women gain 5 kg of weight during the first three years. On an average, during this period, women gain around 1 kg of weight per year. Aging also contributes to these weight changes. Menopausal changes are risky to the health of women if they are not taken care of.

Obesity during menopause is characterized by increased fat distribution around the abdominals. Waist measurements increase due to deposition of fats around the abdominals due to less estrogen values.

We have learned that abdominal obesity is related to type 2 diabetes mellitus, abnormal lipid profile, hypertension, certain cancers and CVD. Therefore, it is dangerous.

The Reasons for These Changes

Due to aging, there are physiological and behavioral changes. Aging leads to decrease in fat-free mass, which leads to decreased RMR (resting metabolic rate). Aging also leads to decrease in physical activity, which results in decreased energy output. If this is accompanied by increased calorie intake, it results in increased weight gain. Along with aging, hormonal imbalances also cause weight gain. Loss of ovarian function and luteal phase of menstrual cycle also contribute to decreased AMR. The psychological negative changes because of menopause lead to craving for food to overcome depression-like conditions.

Effects of Obesity in Menopausal Women

We discussed that menopause leads to obesity. Obesity at the menopausal age is responsible for various health conditions.

- Arthritis: Obese women have four times the risk of osteoarthritis than non-obese women. Women are more susceptible to arthritis than men.

- Loss of estrogen affects the calcium absorption by bones. The rate of formation of new osteocytes is decreased as compared to the rate of elimination of old osteocytes after menopause. This leads to brittleness and weakness of bones. This leads to 5–10% loss in bone mass every year. If this total bone loss reaches up to 30–40%, then the vertebrae (back bones) get worn out.

The study shows that 45% of menopausal women show osteoporosis (brittleness of bones), 15% of women suffer from osteopenia; 10% women do have osteoporosis but they do not have osteopenia and 30% women do not suffer from either osteopenia or osteoarthritis. Osteoporosis leads to fracture of bone due to any minor accident. Obese women with osteoporosis have a very poor recovery from such fractures in their later age. Metabolic rate and decreased physical activity, with or without increased calorie intake, could easily result in weight gain.

The factor that is most consistently related to weight gain in this age group is decreased physical activity. It is not only strongly related to weight gain but is also related to the loss of fat-free mass and increased body fat observed in post-menopausal women. Moreover, evidence suggests that regular exercise in post-menopausal older women can attenuate the accumulation of adipose tissue in the upper and central body regions.

Breast Cancer

- After menopause, women with obesity have a higher risk of developing breast cancer. In addition, weight gain after menopause may also increase breast cancer risk.

- Women who gain about 45 pounds or more, after the age of 18, are twice as likely to develop breast cancer after menopause than women with no weight gain.

- Before menopause, high BMI has been associated with a decreased risk of the most lethal form of breast cancer, called inflammatory breast cancer (IBC), in women with BMI as low as 26.7, regardless of menopausal status.

- Before menopause, women who are overweight and have breast cancer are likely to have a shorter life span than women with lower BMI.

Endometrial Cancer (EC)

- Women with obesity have three to four times the risk of endometrial cancer than women with lower BMI.

- An estimated 34–56% increased risk can be attributed to obesity.

- Body size is a risk factor for EC regardless of where fat is distributed in the body. Women with obesity and diabetes have a three-fold increase in risk for EC, over and above the risk of obesity.

Cardiovascular Disease (CVD)

- In middle and older age groups, heavier weight is associated with CVD and its risk factors, particularly for women.

Gall Bladder Disease

- Obesity is a well-established predictor of gall bladder disease in women.

- Women with obesity have at least twice the risk of gallstone disease than women of normal weight.

Urinary Stress Incontinence

- Obesity is a well-documented risk factor for the involuntary loss of urine as well as urgency.

- Obesity has been found to be a strong risk factor for women for several urinary symptoms after childbirth.

Stigma and Discrimination

- Women with obesity appear to have much more prejudice and discrimination directed against them than men with obesity.

- Obesity contributes to unemployment of women.

- Women with obesity face significant barriers in establishing and maintaining social relationships in a society that emphasizes thinness as physical attractiveness.

Hormone Replacement Therapy

Use of estrogen-progesterone combination hormone replacement therapy (HRT) is widespread among postmenopausal women. Not only is it being prescribed for women who have undergone oophorectomy or hysterectomy or for symptomatic relief during natural menopause, but it is also given as preventive therapy for cardiovascular disease, osteoporosis and dementia. Despite the popular belief that HRT causes weight gain, available data shows no increase in weight gain in women taking HRT compared to those given a placebo.

The evidence on the effect of HRT on central body fat distribution is somewhat mixed. One trial shows that women in both placebo and active treatment groups experienced an increase in waist circumference, although the increase was greater in the placebo group. Unopposed estrogen was associated with a slight reduction in waist circumference. After controlling for weight, the effect of estrogen on reducing waist circumference disappeared. However, two other studies using more advanced techniques to measure body fat composition and distribution have found HRT to have a protective effect on reducing central adiposity.

Weight loss reverses the complications in perimenopausal age due to obesity. The healthy lifestyle practices described in this book are correct and prescribed treatment for weight reduction.

Things to Remember

Dr. Sumedha Bhosale

- Even if you have not felt the need for exercise till menopause, you must start exercising immediately.

- You can start exercise at any age.

- Gym exercise prevents the loss of fat-free mass.

- Gym exercise improves bone density.

- Gym exercise strengthens the muscles, ligaments and tendons, which help the joints to perform well, especially in the later age.

- Gym exercise improves the body composition.

- You can do the gym exercise at your own pace.

- Walking is a good exercise but it is not the complete exercise.

- Yogasana improves the flexibility but not the strength of muscles and density of bone.

- Get the advice and approval of a physician and a gynecologist for your weight reduction program. Before starting aerobics, get the body conditioned and do the exercise under supervision. Follow the principle 'easy to hard, light to heavy and simple to advanced.'

- Get a screening and health assessment done before starting the exercise.

- Even though you are not obese, the healthy lifestyle prescribed in this book will provide you with a protective umbrella for a long post-menopausal life without troubling conditions.

- Keep yourself engaged and busy, mentally as well as physically. Do not feel lonely. Gather all pertinent information about menopause.

- Do visit our menopause clinic under the guidance of Dr. Sanjay Gupte, Dr. Vaishali and Dr. Parag Biniwale.

Remember you are the backbone of your family and you have to be strong and healthy.

- Menopause is the central period of your life. You have to live the same period of life you lived till today. Life expectancy is increasing. Keeping fit and healthy with the healthy lifestyle prescribed in this book is extremely necessary for the quality of your future life.

- Menopause does not mean cessation of sex. Your sex life generally does not have any age barrier, provided you are physically and mentally fit. Consult the experts and get correct knowledge about menopause. If the need arises, do not hesitate to get psycho counseling for this reason or for any other reason.

- Menopause i.e., cessation of menses, should be looked at as a normal and natural phenomenon, like menarche, menstruation and pregnancy. Do not make a big issue out of it. Treat it as a beginning of a new and mature life.

- Control your emotions, think positive, be creative and enjoy the post-menopausal life.

Chapter 23

Lower Back Pain

Dr. Ashish Babhulkar
D. Orth. DNB. (orth), FRCS (TR.& orth)
Mch (Orth) (Liverpool UK)

Many times, degenerative changes in the lumbar region of the spine lead to lower back pain. Most of the times, the frequent cause of activity limitation, among people under the age of 45, includes pain and muscle spasm in the area of the lumber spine.

This is due to:

- Tight muscles in lower back

- Tight hamstrings

- Poor posture

- Weak muscles of abdominals

- Structural abnormalities

Prolonged rides on motorbikes on rough roads and use of wrong footwear are among the reasons for this, even though they may sound minor. Frequent back ache is due to combination of one or more factors. Lower back health is determined by various fitness factors including:

Cardiovascular endurance: If you do plenty of cardiovascular endurance exercise i.e. aerobic exercise, then it provides the disks in between the vertebrae with nutrients and disposes of undesirable wastes through an elevated blood supply. If one does not perform aerobic exercise, he or she may suffer from premature disk degeneration.

Body composition: If your body composition is good, then you have enough strong muscles for proper back function as well as good support for the vertebrae. A person with extra fat increases the stress on the spine, which in turn increases the pressure on the disk and other vertebral structures.

Lower back flexibility: If you have flexibility i.e. a flexible back, only then you can bend forward fully. Without flexibility in the lower back, forward and lateral movements are disrupted. This places excessive strain on the hamstrings, leading to lower back and hamstring pain.

Hamstring flexibility: The pelvis can be rotated forward and backward in the sitting position due to flexible hamstrings. Without flexibility, the above movements get restricted, leading to posterior tilt. This causes disk compression.

Hip flexor flexibility: A person with good flexibility in the hip flexors can achieve a neutral pelvic position. Tight hip flexors exaggerate the anterior pelvic tilt and disk compression.

Abdominal strength/endurance: Strong abdominal muscles contribute greatly in maintaining proper pelvic position. Weak muscles get fatigued. This leads to a strain on the extensor muscles on the back.

Back extensor or spine erector muscles strength: These muscles of the lower back provide stability for the spine to maintain an erect posture and control forward bending. Weak muscles increase the stress on the spine and cause increased disk compression. For proper knowledge of muscles, refer to the muscles charts on page __.

Preventing Lower Back Pain

In addition to doing a regular strength and conditioning program for the appropriate musculature, lower back pain can be combated by maintaining good posture at all times. You can practice the following common everyday tips to avoid the occurrence of lower back pain.

Standing and Walking

Stand with the lower back erect and as flat as possible. By squeezing the buttocks and sucking in and tensing the abdomen, the lower back is straightened. Walk, stand and sit as tall as possible.

Bend the knees when leaning, for e.g. over the sink. Avoid leaning whenever possible and squat with a straight lower back. Avoid high heeled shoes. They shorten the Achilles tendons and increase **swayback.**

Avoid standing for long periods of time. But if it is necessary, alternate leaning on the left and right feet and if possible, use the bent-knee position, by putting one foot on a stool. This stance flattens the lower back.

When standing, do not lean back and support with the hand. Keep the hands in front of the body and lean slightly forward. When turning to walk from a standing position, move the feet first and then the body. Open doors wide enough to walk through comfortably. Carefully judge the height of footpaths before stepping up or down.

Sitting

Sit in such a way that the lower back is flat or slightly convex, never hunched over.

Sit so that the knees are higher than the hips. This may require a footstool, especially for a short person. Hard seat backs that begin contact with the back, four to six inches above the seat and provide a fat support over the entire lower back area, are preferable.

Do not sit in soft or overstuffed chairs or sofas.

Avoid sitting in swivel chairs or chairs on rollers.

Do not sit with legs out straight on an ottoman or footstool.

Never sit in the same position for prolonged periods, get up and move around at regular intervals.

Driving

Push the front seat forward so that the knees are higher than the hips and the pedals are easily reached without stretching.

Sit back with the back flat; do not lean forward; sit tall. Add a flat backrest if the car seat is soft or if you are traveling for a long distance.

If on a long trip, stop every 30–60 minutes. Get out of the car and walk around, tensing the buttocks and abdomen to flatten the back, for several minutes.

Always fasten the seatbelt and shoulder harness. Be sure the car has a properly adjusted headrest.

Lying Down

Sleep or rest only on a flat, firm mattress. If it is not available, place a plywood bed board, not less than three-quarters of an inch thick under the mattress. A thinner board will sag, preventing spine alignment.

When sleeping, the preferred position is on the side, both arms in front, the knees slightly drawn up to the chest. Do not sleep on the stomach.

When lying on the back, place a pillow under the knees; raising the legs flattens the lower back curve.

When lying in bed, do not extend the arms above the head; relax them at the sides.

If the doctor prescribes absolute bedrest, do stay in bed. Raising the body or twisting and turning can strain the back.

Sleep alone or in an oversized bed.

When getting out of bed, turn over on your side, draw up your knees, and then swing your legs over the side of the bed.

Lifting

When lifting, let the legs do the work, using the large muscles of the thighs instead of the smaller muscles of the back. You can achieve this by bending the knees while lifting.

Do not twist the body, face the object. Never lift with the legs straight

Do not lift heavy objects from car trunks. Do not lift from a bending-forward position.

Do not reach over furniture to open and close windows. Tuck in the buttocks and pull in the abdomen when lifting.

Always lift objects by holding them close to the body. Lift heavy load not higher than the waist and a light load not higher than the shoulders, as greater height increases swayback.

To turn while lifting, pivot the feet, and turn the whole body at one time.

Word of Caution

Dr. Sumedha Bhosle

Word of caution during gym exercise:

Be aware of proper form and alignment.

Always maintain a pelvic-neutral alignment and an erect torso during any exercise movements.

Avoid head-forward movement in which the chin is tilted up. When leaning forward, lifting or lowering weights, dumbbells or barbells, always bend at the knees.

Avoid hyper-extending the spine in an unsupported position. Adequate warm-up and cool-own period should be allowed during all exercise classes.

It is important to improve muscle strength and flexibility of all laxed muscles causing back pain, mainly hamstrings and abdomen muscles.

Avoid exercises that may aggravate the condition, such as:

* standing shoulders press

* sit-ups with straight legs

* lift-up with straight legs

* both legs raised straight

* standing or sitting, toe touches, with straight legs

Chapter 24

Obesity, Osteoarthritis and Knee Joint

Dr. Sachin Tapasvi
M.S. (orth), DNB. (orth), M.N.A.M.S.
A. F. A.O. A. (Australia)

Knee joint pain, due to osteoarthritis, after the age of 40, is one of the major complaints of obese persons.

Actually, any joint pain is bad but the knee joint pain leads to restriction on every routine physical activity, like the simple movements of the body, walking, sitting and getting up. You may have to face many hurdles in day-to-day activity due to pain in the knee joint. It takes a longer duration to get rid of knee joint pain. And once the degenerative process starts, it is extremely difficult to halt the same. If you want to be mobile in your later age, you have to prevent your knee joint degeneration.

An obese person has almost four times the risk of osteoarthritis compared to a non-obese person. Weight reduction eases the physical burden on the joints and the chance of developing osteoarthritis attenuates. For overweight persons, reducing 2 units of BMI yields a 60% reduction in the risk for symptomatic osteoarthritis.

Reasons for Knee Joint Pain

Due to Aging

We start using our knee joint when we learn to stand. From that moment, we continuously use the knee joints throughout our life, except when we are immobile. This leads to wearing out of hyaline cartilage, which covers the bone ends.

If you are obese, then it causes additional weight on the knee joints and the degeneration procedure starts earlier. Due to such degeneration, the bone ends become rough. This leads to friction during movement, which is extremely painful. The loss of this protective layer leads to exposure of the inner surface of bone ends, leading to pain. Friction of the exposed bone ends lead to formation of debris. For the absorption of debris, the amount of fluid in the joints, which is known as 'synovial fluid,' increases. This leads to swelling of the knee joints. We say that water has accumulated in the knee joints.

Misconception about Synovial Fluid

Many people feel that, due to aging, the secretion of the lubricating substance, synovial fluid, in the knee joints reduces. They feel this is the reason that makes the knee joints immobile. This is a very wrong concept.

Actually, aging leads to roughness of bones and their friction on each other leads to noise due to grinding during movements, not lack of synovial fluid or oil as they think. This leads to tremendous pain during every movement and immobilization of the joints. The belief that the grinding noise during movement is due to the lack of synovial fluid is an immature and unscientific one. Many people feel that, in order to avoid the grinding noise, they have to increase the intake of fats like ghee, coconut oil or castor oil, as if they are treating rusted hinges! Such intake of additional fats every day is not only a joke but is also dangerous to your health.

Many times, the degenerative changes are more on one side than the other. Generally, the medial side of the knee joint shows more degeneration than the lateral side. This leads to imbalance in the knee joints and they bend. The medial portion of the knee joint has to bear the total weight, which leads to more pain at the site. This leads to further wear and tear at the same site, which results in a condition known as 'bow leg' or 'genu virum.' Very rarely, the opposite situation takes place where the lateral portion of the knee joints wears away. This leads to a condition known as 'knock-knee' or 'genu valgum.'

Symptoms of Knee Joint Osteoarthritis

- You may feel pain in the knee joints after overexertion in the primary stage.

- The pain progresses during the normal use of joints.

- You need the support of a hand while getting up from the sitting position from the floor.

- You may experience a feeling of heaviness in the knee joints during early morning, when you get up from the bed. As you start with your daily routine, you feel the light sensation again.

- In the next stage, pain occurs often. Even a small movement causes pain and it takes a lot of time feel relief from the pain. One tends to be immobile and avoids squatting (during the use of Indian toilets). If there is no alternative, then one needs the support of the hand while getting up. One reduces the speed of walking. There is a continuous feeling of heaviness and swelling in the knee joints.

- In an advanced stage, the bending of the knee joints increases. This leads to increase in the distance between the two knees. It changes the style of walking and one has to oscillate the body on either side.

Treatment

Prevention: Keep your weight proportionate to your height.

- If you are obese or overweight, reduce your weight as early as possible. Accept the healthy lifestyle prescribed in this book.

- During weight reduction, avoid high-impact activities like walking, running and jogging. Remember that hill climbing is contraindicated if you are obese. Even though you are not suffering from osteoarthritis but if you are obese, you exert your knee joints during ascending and descending over the hills. When this happens, you become responsible for your future osteo-arthritic condition. Even brisk walking and aerobic classes on a hard surface are dangerous to the knee joint. If you want to participate in an aerobics class, be sure that the floor surface is shock-absorbing. You must use good shoes. Even during walking, you should use shoes that are as per the following norms.

Norms for the Buying Shoes

- While buying shoes, take care that they are light in weight. Light shoes do not exert additional weight on the ankle joints.

- The sole of the shoes should have a good shock-absorption capacity.

- The shoes should be flexible to take the shape of your feet. This avoids adjustment of your feet to the shape of the shoes.

- Simple shoes without a good sole do not indicate their suitability during exercise, though they may be touted to give you fitness.

Many obese people are under the impression that they can lose their excess weight easily if they start exercising like young children. They become overactive and start jogging, skipping and hill climbing. Such activities exert extra load on the weight-bearing joints, especially the knee joints. Your knee has to bear three times your body weight during every step on the ground. If you do a high-impact activity, then this load increases by 10 times. Now, the total weight your knee joints is equal to your body weight × 3 × 9.8 (gravitational force). This leads to degeneration of the knee joints at a faster rate. It exerts additional load on your other bones e.g. tibia and other joints e.g. ankles, hip joints and lower back. Therefore, it is extremely important to take care of these joints by following scientific weight reduction through a healthy lifestyle.

Regular Exercise to Strengthen and Align the Muscles around Knee Joints

Dr. Sumedha Bhosale

Curative Treatment of Osteoarthritis of Knee Joints

- Orthopedic consultants advise painkillers and antiinflammatory drugs in the first phase.

- You may try physiotherapy exercises to strengthen the muscles surrounding the knee joints.

- Surgery is the last resort.

- Adopt a healthy lifestyle to prevent knee joint osteoarthritis and to avoid surgery. If surgery is unavoidable, then protect the newly replaced joint.

Things to Remember

- Do not allow your weight to rise above normal.

- If there is extra weight, lose it immediately.

- Scientifically strengthen your muscles.

- Gym exercises strengthen the muscles. Stretch them regularly.

- Exercise is an extremely important aspect of life from the point of view of arthritis.

- Weight reduction is important to prevent and treat osteoarthritis.

- Weight reduction is important to protect replaced knee joints after surgery.

A healthy lifestyle is the only treatment for the health of your knees.

Chapter 25

Childhood Obesity

Dr. Vaman Khadilkar
MD, DNB, MRCP (U), DCH (London)
Pediatric and adolescent endocrinologist,
Jehangir hospital, Pune and Bombay Hospital, Mumbai

The World Health Organization has declared obesity as one of the most neglected diseases of significant public health importance in this century. In the United States, there is a great prevalence of overweight and obese children and adolescents. The incidence of obesity at all ages is on the rise in developing countries, including India. In a study done, in 1993 in Mumbai, the incidence of obesity in adults was found to be as high as 30–40%. In the recent times, rising incidence of childhood obesity has been reported from many parts of urban India, such as Pune, Chennai and Delhi. Not only is the incidence of obesity in childhood rising but it is also being seen at an increasingly younger age each year.

Children have a higher proportion of body fat in the first two years of their life. After this age, as they become more active, this fat is lost and they remain relatively thin until about 6–7 years of age. At the age of 6–8 years in girls and 8–10 years in boys, there is a natural phenomenon of regaining body fat. This is nature's way of storing energy for the pubertal growth spurt. This is known as adiposity rebound. Adiposity rebound is much more pronounced in today's children and is also being observed at a younger age. This is a dangerous sign for the onset of obesity.

Etiology of Childhood Obesity

Obesity is a multi-factorial disease that is caused by errors in body energy regulation. The development and maintenance of obesity can be considered to result from the accumulation of small errors in energy balance every day, over several months and years.

Roles of Genes

The genetic makeup of human beings, which reflects a long history of relative scarcity of food, has run into an age of excessive food and calories, and many people cannot readily adapt to this. The increasing rates of obesity cannot be explained by changes in the gene pool. The sudden epidemic of obesity seen worldwide is a result of nutritional excess and not genetic defects. However, it is true that genetic variants that were previously 'silent' are now being triggered by the high availability of energy and fat-dense foods and the increasingly sedentary lifestyle of modern societies. But these can only explain the variation in the severity of obesity. By itself, it cannot explain the sudden global rise in obesity.

Roles of Environment

The rapid increase in the prevalence of obesity emphasizes the role of environmental factors, because genetic changes could not occur at this speed. In the modern world, there is a high-fat diet and low levels of activity. Diverging trends of decreasing energy intake and increasing body weight suggest that reduced physical activity may be the most important causative factor in the initiation and maintenance of obesity. Individual variations in resting energy expenditure exist but by themselves they are unlikely to explain the onset and maintenance of obesity. Sedentary lifestyle, lack of physical activity and television viewing are strongly associated with obesity in children.

A specific problem faced by Indian children is long school hours followed by many hours of tuition classes and the time spent in traveling. This is then followed by homework, which is also prolonged. At the end of this, many families find it very hard to send their children out for any physical activity. This encourages a sedentary lifestyle from the beginning. Thus, obesity in childhood seems to be caused by a combination of environmental factors, sedentary lifestyle and unmasking of some genetic traits due to constant positive energy balance.

The Crucial Periods

Three crucial periods in childhood determine the chance of persistent obesity during adulthood. These periods are:

- Gestational period: Infants of diabetic mothers have a higher chance of becoming obese at 6–10 years and this persists into adulthood.

- Adiposity rebound: Early adiposity rebound is related to parental obesity and persistence of obesity in adulthood.

- Adolescent period: Children who become obese in adolescence have a higher chance of becoming obese adults.

Psychological Causes

Obese children often have psychosocial problems within their families. Insecure children tend to overeat, as food is their solace, thus leading to compulsive eating and obesity. Marital discord, school problems or loss of a very close relative can cause insecurity in the child. In a world where there are increasing demands over children, psychosocial causes of obesity are not uncommon.

Genetic Syndromes

Certain genetic syndromes such as Prader Willi syndrome, Lawrence Moon Biedel syndrome, Cohen and Alstrom syndrome are associated with severe obesity. Children with leptin (a hormone that controls appetite) deficiency become morbidly obese. These syndromes are very rare and form only a very small proportion of obese children.

Children with Challenges

Children with physical challenges and mental sub-normality, who are wheelchair-bound or less mobile, tend to become obese due to lack of physical activity.

Endocrine Obesity

Endocrine obesity (obesity caused by hormonal disorders) is rare in childhood, the incidence being less than 1%. The causes of endocrine obesity are thyroid hormone deficiency and disorders of adrenal and pituitary glands. Children with hormonal disorders that lead to obesity are short and obese, whereas children who have simple or nutritional obesity are tall and obese. This difference is useful for doctors to distinguish between endocrine and non-endocrine obesity.

Recognizing Childhood Obesity

Early detection of childhood obesity is critical because, in the early stage, it is reversible and complications can be prevented. Well-established obesity is frustrating to treat. Every child must have a growth chart, which is routinely updated from birth to 18 years of life. Pediatricians should monitor growth in terms of height and weight on a regular basis. When a child crosses two major percentile lines (3, 10, 25, 50, 75, 90, 97) on the weight chart (upward trend of weight gain), immediate action should be taken to prevent further obesity. It is inappropriate to wait until the child's weight crosses the 85th percentile. At that stage, it can be too late.

Body Mass Index (BMI) Charts

In adulthood, there are fixed BMI cut-off points to define the grade of obesity such as 25 for overweight and 30 for obese. In children, however, there are no such cut-off values. Hence, BMI charts, which are age- and sex-specific, should be used. In India, BMI standards by Agarwal, which were recently adopted by the Indian Academy of Pediatrics, should be used.

Physical Effects of Childhood Obesity

Fat tissue is a hormone-producing organ by itself

Fat tissue, which was once thought to be an inactive store of energy, is now found to be a metabolically very active tissue. By itself, fat is a hormone-producing organ. Fat in the abdomen is the metabolically most active fat. Hence, children with central obesity are at the highest risk of hormonal abnormalities as a result of obesity. Indian children and adolescents do tend to have a higher central obesity with higher abdominal fat, leading to secondary hormonal disorders.

Obesity Related Co-morbidity

Physical effects of childhood obesity are far-reaching and can be devastating over the years. Obesity-associated co-morbidity in children includes significantly increased risks for diabetes, cardiovascular disease, high blood pressure and stroke. It is also observed that children with obesity have a higher incidence of certain cancers. They are also likely to suffer from respiratory diseases such as bronchial asthma, snoring and sleep apnea. Due to excessive weight on the joints, degenerative joint diseases, knocked knees and leg bowing are common. Obesity shortens life span through co-morbidity. So, earlier the onset of obesity, the worse is the prognosis.

Secondary Hormonal Changes Caused By Obesity

Polycystic ovary syndrome (PCOS) is a condition that leads to irregularity of menses, unwanted body hair growth and infertility. This is more commonly seen in obese adolescent girls. A lot of boys with obesity have small genitalia. Most of these have buried genitals rather than true micro genitals. Breast development is seen more commonly in obese boys because of fat deposition in the chest area and also because of increased production of female hormones in the fat tissue.

Childhood obesity is associated with much worse long-term prognosis. Obese children have 2.5 times risk of having high blood pressure and 8.5 times risk of being hypertensive adults.

Fetal Origin of Adult Disease Hypothesis, Childhood Obesity and Its Relevance to India

David Barker and colleagues have shown that if a child is born with growth retardation and later gains excessive weight, he or she is likely to suffer from type 2 diabetes, hypertension, cardiovascular morbidity and stroke, the major killers in adults. In India, there is a high incidence of intrauterine growth retardation (IUGR). And now, on top of this, children are becoming obese leading to a high chance that these major killers mentioned above may affect the younger population. Thus, childhood obesity in the background of IUGR assumes a greater significance in India.

Emotional Problems Caused By Childhood Obesity

Depression, anxiety, and discrimination, both in social life and in the workplace, along with poor self-esteem are common in obese children and adolescents.

Management of Childhood Obesity

Evaluation of Obese Children

Obesity is usually diagnosed by visual impression alone and confirmed by anthropometric parameters and indices plotted on appropriate growth charts. While evaluating obese children, the detailed family history of obesity, hypertension, diabetes and heart disease should be obtained. A detailed diet history and psychological assessment must also performed be done. The family is asked to keep a detailed diary of the diet and physical activity of the child.

1. Body mass index (BMI) should be calculated using the formula: weight in kg/height in meters

2. BMI should be plotted on age- and sex-specific BMI charts, and the severity of obesity should be determined. Any child above the 85th percentile for age and sex is overweight and above the 95th percentile is obese. A detailed clinical examination should be done. Blood pressure should be measured.

Investigations

Investigations of an obese child or adolescent include measurement of lipid profile, blood sugar, liver function tests, respiratory function tests and sleep studies. Thyroid function tests are also done.

Basic Principles of Management

The mainstay of treatment of obesity in childhood is diet and exercise. A diet low in calorie and fat and high in fiber is recommended. The basic goal should be reduction in energy intake and increase in energy expenditure. Increase in physical activity is also recommended, with regular aerobic exercise. Reduction in television viewing and computer games is insisted upon. Children are encouraged to play outdoors and not within their homes.

An Indian Approach to Diet Is as Follows

Half of the meal should consist of salads, vegetables and fruits, quarter must be proteins e.g. milk, egg, dal, and the remaining quarter must comprise complex carbohydrates such as rice and chapati.

Goal of Management

1. **Medical:** Resolution of complications and co-morbidity

2. **Behavioral:** Achieve healthy eating habits and active lifestyle, instead of focusing on ideal body weight. Care should be taken to avoid nutritional deficiencies while planning diet.

Prevention of Obesity

Obesity is a very frustrating disorder to treat for the family as well as for the physician. It is therefore critical that it is prevented. Health education starting from pregnancy throughout childhood is important and the pediatrician has an important role to play. Growth monitoring is the key for early detection of obesity. Whenever a child shows an upward movement of more than two percentile lines on a weight chart within 6 months to 1 year, it should be noted seriously and parental education with change in the lifestyle for the family must be advocated.

Approach for prevention is age-specific. In infancy, parent education should center on promotion of breastfeeding, recognition of signals of satiety and delayed introduction of solid foods. In childhood and adolescence, it should focus on proper nutrition, selection of low-fat snacks, good exercise, activities and habits, and monitoring of television viewing. Overall sedentary behavior should be reduced.

Wider-scale efforts to prevent and treat childhood obesity should include recreational opportunities for children, changes in housing and neighborhoods, and changes in the macro environment, such as proper food marketing, transport systems, urban planning and behavior change involving the whole family and society at large.

Medications

Medications for the treatment of obesity is not routinely recommended in children or adolescents. Anti-obesity drugs are not approved for long-term use in youth. They have not been extensively tested for safety over long periods of time; they may only benefit a minority of patients and may be associated with serious cardiovascular side effects.

The major groups of drugs are (a) those that reduce food intake e.g. monoamine oxidase inhibitors and sympathomimetic drugs (b) those that increase energy expenditure e.g. ephedrine and caffeine and (c) those that inhibit fat absorption.

The use of agents to induce dietary fat malabsorption is associated with significant intestinal discomfort, flatulence and social embarrassment.

Metformin, an anti-diabetic medication, has shown promise in helping obese patients adhere to a diet and maintain better weight control. This agent is particularly promising in the Indian context as Indian children are prone to diabetes because of genetic susceptibility, which is further aggravated by obesity.

Medications are used in children only when they have other associated risk factors such as diabetes or high blood pressure.

Intensive Diet

Diets such as protein-sparing modified fast, which gives adequate amount of protein but severely restricts the calories (2400–3360 K joule per day), were popular for a few years but they are not physiological and lead to complications such as liver problems and diarrhea. It cannot be given beyond 12 weeks. Although they are useful in short-term weight loss, they are not superior in maintenance of reduced weight when compared to diet, exercise and lifestyle change. This type of diet is not particularly useful in childhood obesity. In India, this kind of diet is not easily available and should best be kept as a last resort in adolescents.

Behavior Modification Program

Behavior modification approaches are used to help patients make long-term changes in their eating and exercise behavior. Behavioral approaches stress on monitoring of dietary intake, physical activity, self-monitoring and stimulus control. Behavior modification also includes changing the act of eating, increasing the motivation, managing stress and prevention of relapse. Better results have been achieved in behavioral programs that provide longer periods of treatment contact, more structured approaches to modifying dietary intake and higher goals for physical activity.

Weight-Loss Surgery

Surgical procedures, which are undertaken in the management of obesity, are mainly to reduce the fat mass. These include methods such as liposuction, which is purely cosmetic, and procedures to reduce the absorption of nutrients from the gastrointestinal tract. These procedures together are called 'bariatric surgery.' These are associated with significant weight loss and complications such as liver problems, malabsorption, iron and folate deficiency, and small bowel obstruction. The surgery is recommended in only those patients who are in the adolescent age group with morbid obesity (BMI above 40) and an associated complication, such as diabetes. Bariatric surgery is the last resort when medical management has completely failed.

Conclusion

Obesity in children is a rapidly growing problem worldwide, including India, especially urban India. It has devastating long-term consequences. Childhood obesity should be diagnosed using BMI charts specifically designed for this population. It is far more devastating than adult obesity. Earlier is the age of onset of obesity, worse is the prognosis. India has very large number of babies born with growth retardation. In the context of fetal origin of adult disease hypothesis, IUGR adds another dimension to the problem of obesity in India. Obesity is a very difficult and frustrating disease to treat when it is well established. Therefore, all efforts must be directed at recognizing and preventing obesity early in life. Pediatricians have a critical role to play in the prevention of obesity in childhood.

Chapter 26

Osteoarthritis

Dr. Ashish Bhabhulkar
D. (orth) DNB (orth) FRCS (Tr and Orth)
M.C.H. (orth) (Liverpool UK)

Osteoarthritis is a degenerative joint disease. Joints link bones together. They form a functional unit that causes body movement. It is a place of contact or connection between the bones and cartilage. Cartilage is the gristly tissue that covers the ends of the bones. It helps in absorbing the impact and friction of bones that bump and rub against each other.

The presence of cartilage at the bone ends helps avoid friction during movement by facilitating smooth joint movement. A gradual wearing of this protective hyaline cartilage leads to osteoarthritis. Osteoarthritis is the most common form of arthritis. Nearly everyone gets stricken by it, sooner or later. It rarely begins before the age of 45. It develops gradually. Initially, it is restricted to only one or a few joints. Almost any joint may be affected but generally the joints in spine, hips and legs are affected. In women, the fingers are particularly affected. Involvement of the hip joint and knee joint is common. After the age of 60, it can become increasingly troublesome and occasionally disabling. Osteoarthritis in spine may be quite severe but it does not show any symptoms.

Osteoarthritis involves damage to the cartilage. The exact cause of osteoarthritis is not known but obesity creates further strain on weakened joints. Many acute sports injuries cause such cartilage damage. Repetitive low-grade impact leads to bumping and grinding of the cartilage.

Symptoms of Osteoarthritis

- Pain after exercise

- Restricted range of movement, stiffness after activity

- Swelling

- Warm sensation

- All the above are signs of inflammation

- As the condition progresses, movements become more and more restricted

- Troublesome soreness

- Grating sensation while moving the joints and immobility in severe cases

Treatment of Osteoarthritis Is Entirely Palliative

Weight reduction is the first important part of treatment. It prevents further damage. In day-to-day activity, your weight-bearing joints viz. hip joints, knee joints and ankle joints have to bear the weight, which is three times more during the simple movements of sitting, standing, ascending and descending staircases. Every extra kilo of additional weight results in almost 3 kg of additional weight on these weight-bearing joints. Therefore, reduction in weight by 10 kg reduces 30 kg of weight on each joint, during each movement described above.

In obese patients with osteoarthritis, it is extremely important to lose weight to protect the joint from further and fast damage due to wear and tear.

Role of Exercise in Arthritic Clients

Dr. Sumedha Bhosale

- Exercise helps preserve strength and joint mobility.

- It improves functional capabilities.

- It relieves pain and stiffness.

- It prevents further deformities.

- It re-establishes neuro-muscular coordination.

- It mobilizes stiff and contracted joints.

- It improves overall physical conditioning.

Sample Exercise Program

Mode – Non-weight-bearing activities such as cycling, swimming as they reduce further joint stress

Intensity – Low and based on pain-tolerance of clients

Frequency – At least 4 to 5 days a week

Duration – Longer and more gradual warm-up and cool-down; greater than 10 minutes; total exercise duration depending on clients' capacity

Word of Caution

- Avoid exercise during acute stage, as fatigue is a common complaint to be noticed.

- Ensure adequate rest between two sets of exercise.

- Ensure extended warm-up to promote flexibility and range of motion.

- Exercise with mild or moderate intensity and slow speed, with good control.

- Avoid excessive movement such as low-impact exercise.

- Begin with low intensity and frequent rest.

- Stretch the portion of the exercise to focus on the arthritic joint.

- If you are unable to do other exercises, cycling or swimming is preferred.

- The posture must be correct to avoid fatigue and joint stress. Proper body alignment is very important.

- During exercise, the joint is supposed to be in the most stable and functional position.

- Gym exercises are to be performed using light weights to increase muscle strength and endurance without any other joint movements.

- Accept your own limitations and plan accordingly, with the help of a health counselor and as per the guidelines of your orthopedic consultant.

- Ensure you take sufficient rest.

The diet should be as per the guidelines of your dietician. Weight reduction is extremely important. If you are obese, you have 40% more chance to develop osteoarthritis.

Chapter 27

Obesity and Sex Life

A rewarding sex life is one of the ingredients of a continuing sense of wellbeing. While everyone has a potential for a healthy and fulfilling sex life, developing it and maintaining it is important. Many times, problems arise in sexual life and it becomes difficult to deal with them.

Obesity often leads to sexual problems. Obese males may experience impotence due to increased weight. The blood vessels supplying blood to the sex organs get clogged due to atherosclerosis. Hampered blood supply leads to impotence.

Psychological reasons like shame, low self-esteem and lack of confidence also lead to impotence. Obese persons may experience depression, poor sex performance, poor sexual response, feeling of guilt, insecurity about techniques and inferiority complex. Stress from all these issues may spill over into the relationship.

Women are more sensitive than men. Problems like frigidity are very common in obese women. This results in depression, leading to weight gain, further poor performance, increased guilt and increased inferiority complex, which altogether lead to further weight gain.

Weight reduction helps improve sexual behavior. A weight-reduction program gives you beauty and confidence along with good health. The blood lipid profile improves. Blood circulation all over the body also improves.

Gym exercise improves hormonal metabolism. The level of testosterone is directly related to improved performance. The libido returns. You can please your partner and get pleasure from your partner. This improves your self-esteem and you tend to stick to your weight reduction program. Then you find a new person within yourself.

In case you are extremely obese and it is a long journey to reach your 'realistic targeted normal weight,' even a small weight reduction of 10% due to exercise improves your sex performance. You have to learn to cope up with your physical status and enjoy your sex life.

Knowledge and understanding the physiology and techniques of sex life, with the help of a consultant, care and efforts for yourself and from your partner, understanding each other's emotions, respecting each other, learning various techniques that are not only physical but are psychological too, love and respect for each other, encouraging the partner for weight reduction, and a caring attitude will help you achieve a happy and fulfilling sex life. Thus, your quality of life improves.

Chapter 28

Coping with Obesity

Dr. Lily Joshi
M.D. (medicine)

One of the most painful aspects of obesity may be the emotional suffering it can cause. Being slim is generally associated with good health, beauty and success. Whereas obese people are generally viewed upon a lazy, gluttons or lacking in will power. This brings feelings of guilt, shame, frustration and depression among the obese.

Obesity should be viewed as a chronic disease condition and not a moral failing or a personal choice. Obese people need to cultivate a positive attitude toward their condition. They should take charge of their own status and resolve to make a good therapeutic plan to shed those extra kilos (5–10% of their weight) and try sincerely. Then success will be theirs!

– Dr. Lily Joshi

Coping with Obesity

Dr. Sumedha Bhosale

We learned from the previous chapter that we have to cultivate a positive attitude toward the condition we are suffering from. We also have to avoid miracle treatments. We have to change our mindset toward obesity.

You know your condition is a complex phenomenon of your physiology, psychology and genetics. You have learned about the treatment. You have changed your lifestyle. You are going to achieve your realistic weight and maintain it.

- Exercise as per your capacity. Do not over-exercise or under-exercise.

- If you get tempted to eat any food that you are not supposed to eat, then try it at breakfast time. Have your prescribed breakfast i.e. 2 servings of salads and 1 serving of protein. Instead of two servings of complex carbohydrate, you may have 2–3 teaspoons of your favorite sweet preparation, a very small portion of the food that is the cause of your temptation. Then follow your prescribed low-cal diet for the rest of the day.

- In case there is any slip, do not feel guilty afterwards. Do not skip any meal or do not exercise for more than one hour. Follow your planned diet from the next day.

- Do not hesitate to wear the clothes you like.

- Just ignore the ridiculous comments from any one around you. It is their lack of knowledge about your condition. Just overlook such things. Enjoy life. Life is full of so many joyous things. Take pleasure from these things.

- Strengthen your mind. Take support from a support group. Help other obese individuals make up their minds.

- The world is full of variety. Some of us are underweight, some of us are overweight, and some of us have other medical conditions. Everybody has their own problem. Obesity is one such problem. Let it not affect your life as you have started the treatment.

- You are losing weight to prevent diseases. Your obesity should not affect your self-esteem. Inner beauty is important. You must grow it by having a healthy body, a healthy mind and a healthy attitude. Inner beauty lasts forever even when you grow older. Positive self-acceptance is an extremely important aspect of your life. The society needs to focus on health and wellness instead of the body size.

Take the initiative to build such a society.

Throw away shame, guilt, frustration and depression. Accept a healthy lifestyle. Build a healthy mind. Build a healthy society. It is your responsibility to help other obese people build their health. Be healthy and be happy!

Chapter 29

Obesity and Medicines

Dr. Shrirang Godbole

M.D. (med.), DNB (endocrinology)

Many times, during the weight-reduction program, in spite of proper calorie control and scientific exercise, the rate of weight reduction is not up to the mark. You may get disturbed mentally. We have learned that the phenomenon of obesity is complex and there are many chemicals controlling obesity. During this juncture, when your efforts are not paying off, you have to consult your physician. The physician may prescribe some medication for obesity.

You have to remember that only drugs are not effective at all. They are proven to be effective only if you stick to a healthy lifestyle, as prescribed in this book. After discontinuing any of the aspect of a healthy lifestyle, you regain the lost weight immediately, even though you are under medication.

In the market, there are many off-label pharmaceutical agents and you may get tempted to use their products on your own. Many clinicians too prescribe them. These drugs give only psychological help to stick to a healthy lifestyle. But whatever you lose is because of exercise and calorie control.

From a practical standpoint, it is important to recognize that medication can contribute to improved results only among certain patients.

- **Sibutramine:** If the body mass index is above 30 or if you are having any medical problem and your BMI is above 27, then this drug is recommended. It affects satiety and improves metabolic rate. It should not be used if you have renal (kidney) impairment, dialysis and liver diseases. Sibutramine provides the benefits of reduction in serum uric acid and serum cholesterol.

  ➤ **Orlistat:** This drug inhibits the action of lipase enzyme, which digests fat. One has to control calories when this drug is prescribed. It is a first drug in a new class. It blocks the absorption of dietary fats. It can be prescribed to adolescents of ages 12 to 16 years. It inactivates the enzymes that digest the fats. As a result, less fat is absorbed by the body and calorie intake is further restricted. This results in creation of negative energy balance, which leads to weight reduction. About 30% of the fat is prevented from getting absorbed.

> ➤ **Rimonabant:** It suppresses the appetite by inhibiting the receptors found in the system. It plays a key role in the regulation of central and peripheral energy balance, glucose balance and lipid balance. Excessive food intake results in over-activeness of the system. This over-activeness triggers a cycle of increased eating, fat storage and obesity. Rimonabant appears to modulate food intake i.e. suppresses appetite. This drug controls tobacco dependency as well. It may produce side effects like depression, nausea, vomiting, diarrhea, headache, dizziness and anxiety. Sometimes, it causes sleep disturbances and suicidal ideation.

In June 2007, an endocrinological and metabolic advisory committee voted unanimously against the approval of rimonabant for treatment of weight loss for the above-mentioned serious psychiatric side effects. A final decision on this is awaited.

- **Metformin** is an anti-diabetic drug for type 11 diabetes. It sensitizes insulin that enhances glucose uptake without promoting insulin secretion. The Food and Drug Association has not approved it as a weight loss agent but it is used by some practitioners for obesity.

- **Topiramate and Zonisamide:** Actually, they were used to treat seizure. Incidentally, they were found to help in losing weight.

  > ➤ **Bupropion:** It is prescribed for treatment of depression and tobacco cessation. Its role in weight reduction is not clear but it regulates food intake. The common side effects are agitation, dry mouth, insomnia (sleeplessness), headache/migraine, nausea/vomiting, constipation and tremor.

- **Fluoxetine:** It is commonly used to treat depression, binge eating and purging behavior in bulimia nervosa.

Some medications act on the satiety center of the brain. Phentermine, diethylpropion, benzphetamine and phendimetrazine suppress appetite and later increase energy expenditure. Mazindol stimulates thermogenesis and possibly delays gastric emptying. Most of these drugs are associated with abuse, particularly in long-term use. When tolerance develops, the dosage should not be exceeded in an attempt to restore effect. The drug should be discontinued. When medications for weight loss are stopped, in a few months, all the weight that has been lost is gradually regained.

There are some over-the-counter diet products that promise to help you shed your excess weight, by either suppressing your appetite or raising the metabolic rate.

Caffeine has the ability to enhance mobilization of fatty acids and thus conserve glycogen stores. Caffeine may also directly affect muscle contractility, possibly by facilitating calcium transport. It reduces plasma K+ accumulation, which is responsible for muscle fatigue.

Caffeine has a diuretic action. This shows less weight due to increased urination but it leads to dehydration. It causes cramps and several other problems related to dehydration, such as electrolyte imbalances and cardiac output.

- **Diuretics and laxatives:** Diuretics increase urination and laxatives increase bowel movements, which lead to frequent motions. Both treatments are ineffective for the long term. These treatments also lead to dehydration, followed by electrolyte imbalance and cardiac problems.

- **Chromium:** Chromium picolinate is a mineral needed by the body in minute amounts. It helps the metabolism of blood sugar and blood lipid. Its RDA is 50–200 mg.

Our daily diet fulfills the RDA of chromium picolinate. Therefore, it is not advisable to take them externally. Additional mineral exerts load on kidneys during excretion. It is not found to be useful in losing weight when taken externally.

Garcinia, Sr. John's Wort and 5-Hydroxy-Tryptophan are herbal medicines. The FDA has issued warming regarding pills containing 'Ma.Husang,' like botanical sources, because of many reports of adverse reactions including increased blood pressure, heart rate, heart attack and stroke.

Remember, there is no medicine that has been invented till today, which helps you lose weight even when you are physically inactive and eat whatever you want. Only if you commit yourself to a healthy lifestyle for more than three months and your physician advices you to consume Sibutramine or any other medicine, can you think about medication for weight reduction.

Message from Dr. Sumedha Bhosale

We have learned in detail information related to medical treatment.

1. Even with a drug, you have to follow a healthy lifestyle, otherwise it is futile.

2. Discontinuation of drug leads to regaining lost weight. Continuation may lead to development of tolerance. The drug should be tapered off under medical supervision.

3. Drugs should be used only if it is prescribed by authentic medical experts.

4. The sensible way to lose weight is by practicing control of mind, with an intensive desire to control appetite and overeating. This has to be coupled with exercise to improve thermogenesis.

5. Avoid pharmacological aid unless it is unavoidable and follow a healthy lifestyle.

Chapter 30

Losing Weight the Surgical Way

Dr. Shrihari Dhore Patil
(M.S., F.A.I.S., F.I.C.S.)

In chapter one of this book, you learned about the techniques of measurement of obesity. Let us go through the classification once again.

Overweight and obesity classification by body mass Index (BMI)

National Heart, Lung and Blood Institute Classification BMI (kg/m)

Normal	18.5–24.9
Overweight	25.0–29.9
Obesity class 1	30.0–34.9
Obesity class 2	35.0–39.9
Obesity class 3	(Morbid obesity) = 40.0
Obesity class 3	(Morbid obesity) = 40.0

People who are overweight and obese can be treated successfully through a commitment to a healthy lifestyle. However, morbid obesity is a major challenge. In these cases, surgery is the last choice of treatment.

In chapter two, we saw how obesity matters. Extreme obesity rarely responds to conservative regimens. Therefore, the patient has to undergo surgery. This specialty surgery is called bariatric surgery (weight loss surgery). It has been proved that bariatric surgery is the only option that gives definitive and permanent weight loss to these people.

Bariatric Operations

There are two types of operations for weight loss.

- Restrictive operations

- Mal-absorptive operations

Restrictive operations make the stomach smaller. The person will feel full more quickly than when his stomach was of its original size. This reduces the amount of food eaten and consequently the calories consumed. This leads to weight loss. The most common restrictive surgery is 'gastric banding.'

Gastric Banding

In this operation, a small band is placed around the upper part of the stomach, creating a small pouch. The small size of the pouch means you feel full sooner. However, the band can be adjusted by inflating or deflating the band. This allows adjusting the size of the opening between the pouch and the stomach.

Gastric banding is associated with a short hospital stay, rapid recovery and less risk of complications. After this operation, the person will be able to eat only 1 cup of food (236.6ml) or less, at a time. Certain rules are to be followed after surgery. One must be careful while chewing food. One must stop eating when they feel full. This can take some adjustment, as they will feel full after eating very little food than they are used to eating. They should not drink while eating; otherwise, the food eaten will be washed down the pouch and the person can eat more than the pouch size. After surgery, one has to avoid sweets to achieve good weight loss. Gastric banding was approved by the US FDA in 2001.

You may expect some problems if everything doesn't go well with the surgery. Problems with this procedure include occasional slippage or migration of the band or development of an excessively large upper gastric pouch with vomiting. Also, the outlet from the upper pouch can be occasionally left too large for adequate gastric restriction and weight loss. Then there is a chance of infection of the band.

Gastric Bypass (Roux-en-Y Gastric Bypass)

Gastric bypass surgery makes the stomach smaller and allows food to bypass a part of the small intestine. Bypassing a part of the intestine results in fewer calories being absorbed. This leads to weight loss. The most common gastric bypass surgery is Roux-en-Y gastric bypass. In normal digestion, food passes through the stomach and enters the small intestine, where most of the nutrients and calories are absorbed. It then passes into the large intestine (colon), and the remaining waste is eventually excreted. In a Roux-en-Y gastric bypass, the stomach is made smaller by creating a small pouch at the top of the stomach using surgical staples or a plastic band. The smaller stomach is connected directly to the middle portion of the small intestine (jejunum), bypassing the rest of the stomach and the upper portion of the small intestine (duodenum).

Gastric Balloons

This type of surgery is used for patients who are otherwise unfit to undergo any other type of surgery. The weight loss is modest, temporary and may lead to some complications.

Bariatric surgical procedures will help severely obese individuals lose weight. They can help reshape the body through cosmetic procedures. But it is important to understand that, many times, surgery can be prevented with a proper dietary regime and a regular exercise program.

Who is suitable for obesity surgery?

- People with severe morbid obesity or (BMl (body mass index) > 40kg/m^2) or severe obesity (BMl > 35kg/m^2) with medical co-morbidities or complications of obesity.

- Those who face failure with significant nonsurgical attempts at weight reduction.

- The patient must fully understand the bariatric surgical concepts, accept the risks involved, undergo pre-operative endocrinological and psychological tests and dietician's evaluation, and give consent after being fully informed.

- The patient must be motivated and willing for lifelong follow-up.

- The patient must be psychologically stable and not be a drug abuser.

- People in the age group of 18–65 years, preferably.

Weight Management After Surgery

Dr. Sumedha Bhosale

Even though surgery effectively helps lose weight, in the long term if you do not commit yourself to a healthy lifestyle, you will again start eating a lot and you will regain the lost weight and more.

- **Liposuction:** It is a cosmetic surgery and not a weight reduction technique because only 2–3 kg of fat can be removed at a time. We do not get the anticipated outcome in all cases.

Conclusion

At this stage, I want to bring to your notice that there is the only one and only one solution for prevention of obesity and treatment of obesity and that is commitment to a healthy lifestyle i.e. a combination of exercise, low-cal nutritious diet, rest and relaxation, and positive mental attitude.

Chapter 31

Testimonials

A Few Words from My Few Symbolic Clients (Representative of Group)

An artist is an athlete philosopher. The word 'athlete' in this saying is related to fitness. There is no alternative to exercise if you want to be fit. There is no alternative to a healthy lifestyle if you want to be healthy. For the last so many years, I have been exercising in Status Health Club.

– Dr. Shriram Lagu

For the last 12 years, I have been a member of Status Health Club. I have lost my extra weight. I am maintaining it and, most importantly, I got rid of my cervical spondylitis. My whole family are members of Status Health Club. Day by day, I am realizing that we are all getting more and more fit. We are enjoying a healthy lifestyle.

– Mrs. Swapna Pednekar,
Owner, Swapnanjali Jewellery Studio

I was pretty impressed by the lecture given by Dr. Sumedha Bhosale about obesity and healthy lifestyle. I asked her if it was possible to lose weight at my age of 78 years and control my diabetes and hypertension with minimum medication. Every day, I used to depend on 14 tablets for my various ailments. I used to think negatively that perhaps I might not witness and enjoy the wedding of my grandson, which recently I myself organized with great enthusiasm. This was possible only because of a weight reduction of 8 kg in the last four months. My dependence on medication has been considerably reduced. I am strongly committed to the healthy lifestyle program prescribed by Dr. Sumedha Bhosale. I am promoting it very enthusiastically among my friends by setting myself as their role model.

– Rotarian Tatya Sapre

My long-cherished dream of motherhood became a reality five years ago. I was suffering from gynecological disorders, for which I was under treatment for more than six years. My gynecologist advised me to lose weight. I registered myself at Status, a medical health club. In the very first discussion with

Dr. Sumedha madam, I became very positive about my dream becoming a reality. She said, "Do not worry at all. Be positive. Don't worry about the exercise. Our instructors will get them done by you. But follow the diet meticulously. Give your 100% efforts and you will definitely get good results. You will realize your dream." She assured me that every year at least four to five patients realize their dream of motherhood. Within a short span of six months, I got very good results. Now I have a wonderful five-year-old daughter, who incidentally loves eating salads. I have reduced my weight after the birth of my daughter and I am maintaining it successfully.

– Pratibha

I am a young diabetic, suffering from knee ligament injury. This put a limitation on my exercise routine. Apart from this, I love to eat. My weight was increasing and causing problems for me. Then I enrolled at Status Health Club. Here, my diabetes came under control, my knee ligament was made better, and my weight was reduced. Here, I found a family, which was very particular about health. I made many new, highly-educated, like-minded friends.

– Alok Telang, entrepreneur

In the marriage scene, everybody wants a fair, good-looking and a slim bride. I was fair and good-looking, but on the weighty side. Many prospective bridegrooms were rejecting me only because I was fat. I was very worried thinking that I might have to settle for a bridegroom who was not of my choice. But then Shilpa aunty convinced me to enroll myself at Status Health Club, where she had successfully reduced her weight. Here I reduced my weight and started getting acceptance from many grooms who were a match to my status. I have now found a suitable life partner for myself. I might even be married before the publication of this book.

– Pooja

At my age of 16, it was very tedious to follow a diet and exercise. Dr. Sumedha madam kept advising me continuously about a nutritious diet. She suggested so many instant recipes like diet *bhel*, diet culets, *masala idli* and so on. My mom used to get angry with me almost every day, for my demand to have variety in my food. I didn't like to have ordinary regular food for dinner. I tried various recipes of salads to make my meals tastier. Now all my family members are enjoying salads. I lost 16 kg and everybody around me is now appreciating my good figure. The most important fact is that my mom has stopped complaining about me. Now we are good friends. And yes, I can wear jeans! Sumedha madam is helping me realize my dream of becoming an aerobics instructor.

– Prajakta Pendse

Sumedha *mavshi* told me that if I took efforts to grow tall by eating proteins and a balanced diet, along with exercises, then it is not necessary for me to lose weight. She allowed only 50% of food from outside. She said that if I ate only at home, then I can grow tall at a fast rate. In the last 6 months, I have gained 3 inches height and my tummy has become flat. I have decided to continue with this height-gain program.

– Tejas Mhalgi (age 11 years)

I am a computer engineer. I work on the PC for 10 hours every day. I had put on 16 kg in four months. I decided to lose my weight and registered with Status club. Dr. Sumedha madam said that during weight reduction we would incorporate exercises that would prevent the spine from getting spondylitis. Within a period of 3 weeks, I realized that Dr. Sumedha had diagnosed my spondylitis, though I had no symptoms. Along with my weight loss, I am reaping the benefits of relaxed shoulders, neck and upper back.

– Anirudha Pujari

I was suffering from arthritis and it was extremely painful for me to walk even 10 steps without pain. With the help of exercises, as per the guidelines of Dr. Sumedha and medication, I successfully overcame this painful condition. The confidence she has generated in me is amazing!

– Jayashree Ramesh Joshi

My instructor made me do the exercises prescribed by Dr. Sumedha madam. I also followed the diet given by her. At the age of 58 years, I lost 11 kg and I am enjoying my new lifestyle.

– Sulabha Gore, well-known vocalist

I feel extremely charged whenever I have a talk with Dr. Sumedha. I try to be regular in my exercises at the gym. If I cannot go to the gym, I exercise at home as per the instructions given by Dr. Sumedha. Whenever I feel exhausted during my meetings, I just call her and get recharged. She provides good tips about protective foods, antioxidants and anti-cancer natural foods. I feel extremely energetic after exchanging a few words with her.

– Mukta Manohar, labor activist

I am very lucky I got a good friend in Dr. Sumedha, with whom I can share anything, at any time. I am losing weight. I got rid of my lower back ache. Whenever I go to America to see my children and grandson, I feel confident that I can successfully complete my duties over there and maintain my fitness at a higher level.

– Usha Akotkar

Dr. Sumedha madam said that if I become an aerobics instructor after weight reduction, I will forget that I used to have asthmatic attacks so frequently. In the last two years, I did not have any asthmatic episode. Even though I wish to disclose my name, she didn't allow me to do so. She said some things are better if they remained confidential. She is extremely concerned about my good future along with my good health.

– Aerobics instructor working out of India

I wanted to lose 7 kg in 5 weeks to get selected in an interview for the position of an airhostess. I lost 7 kg in 5 weeks Dr. Sumedha madam said that I should check my hemoglobin before the weight reduction program. It was 11.5 g. After my weight reduction program, it increased to 12 g. I improved my fitness, lost weight and improved my hemoglobin level.

– Neeru

I was an obese beautician and I registered at Status for my weight reduction program. Dr. Sumedha madam advised me to complete an instructor training program and start a slimming center attached to my parlor. I completed the program and I am now guiding my parlor clients in losing weight too. Before losing my targeted weight, I started promoting a scientific weight reduction program. I am pretty confident that I will lose my last 20 kg in the next 6 months and I can guide my clients as well.

– Shivani Joshi

I was 85 kg after my delivery. I lost 26 kg before the first birthday of my daughter. Now my daughter is 4 years old. I am maintaining my weight. I have also managed to lose 3 kg more. I am enjoying a healthy lifestyle.

– Anjali Deshpande

I was obese. Then I lost 10 kg. I passed an instructor training course at Status and I am now working as a gym-cum-aerobics instructor at Status. I benefited from the magic touch of Dr. Sumedha madam and I am enjoying a healthy lifestyle and experiencing a wonderful life. My personality has changed totally. I can wear all kinds of clothes. I am feeling like a butterfly.

– Deepali Rasker

Dr. Sumedha is an impressive and powerful counselor. My wife changed from within herself. She listened to Sumedha ma'am and has achieved a great level of confidence. On the first day, she climbed the staircase of Status with my support. Within a period of one month, she could climb Jyotiba mountain near Kolhapur with full confidence. Generally, no doctor can impress me but I was amazed when Dr. Sumedha convinced me with a scientific explanation for each food group, with so many options. I am a scientist and I know all the minute details of grains like ragi and oats and sources of selenium and calcium. I was enjoying the theoretical knowledge getting implemented practically. I got enlightened and changed my views and started practicing the knowledge of food, grains and vegetables in my day-to-day practice.

– Dr. Ramchandra Sable
Ph.D. (agronomy, metrology)
Principle of Mahatma Phule
Krishi Veedyapeeth Agriculture College, Pune

I am a beautician at Narayangaon. One day in 2003, I went through an advertisement in the daily *Sakal* about an instructor training course in English and Marathi. I was weak in English but I was very happy because now I could learn this science in Marathi and could start a slimming center adjacent to my parlor in Narayangaon. I was tensed when I enrolled myself for this course. When I attended the first lecture, I was so impressed by the personality of Dr. Sumedha that I decided to score the highest in my batch. She encouraged me a lot. She taught in Marathi and encouraged me to learn the same in English as well. She personally trained me. She not only helped me learn everything but also inaugurated my slimming center in Narayangaon that year in spite of her extremely busy schedule. She supported me strongly in my early career days so that I could treat my first few clients with her consultation over telephone. Slowly, I became independent. She is a sculptor not just a doctor. I respect Dr. Sumedha madam a lot.

– Vrinda Narayangaon

I feel personality matters a lot. When your weight increases, you feel so embarrassed. Others cannot even imagine how you are feeling. You need support, at least from your spouse. Or else, you may end up in depression. The comments from people around you depress you. Due to depression, you start overeating. There are also other medical disorders due to obesity. So many things form a trap, which leads to further weight gain. A vicious circle set in. I too was a victim of such a vicious circle. I was a sportsperson but long ago, on March 8, 2004, on Women's Day, I read about a discount offer for a weight reduction program for women at Status Health Club, I appreciated the idea behind the discount. I was eager to see the person behind this idea. Yes, she was Dr. Sumedha. I was pretty impressed to see her giving assurance to every client while giving information about her discount scheme. Being a woman, she could understand the demands of other women. I enrolled myself in the program. I got something beyond a scientific exercise plan—it is the mental support given by each staff member and Dr. Sumedha. My instructors, receptionists, dietician and Sumedha madam, everybody, saw the change in me. Everybody congratulated me. Dr. Sumedha was very keen to make sure I was not eating lesser than what was prescribed. I didn't realize that I was losing so efficiently that everyone around me was appreciating the changes in my measurements.

It was a great period of achievements and success. I feel my husband rewarded me with a valuable gift—encouragement to enroll at Status. I am grateful to my husband for such a gift and Status Health Club for providing me a new fit family with their staff and clients. I am a proud family member of Status.

– Mrs. Kawade,
union leader,
Bank of Maharashtra

Section V

Wellness

Chapter 32

Wellness

The Don'ts of a Healthy Routine

- Avoid eating simple carbohydrates like sugar, jaggery and honey.

- Avoid deep-fried stuff, junk food, fats, soft drinks and hard drinks.

- Do not munch between meals.

- Do not nap after meals.

- Do not miss exercise at any cost.

- Spend at least one wakeful hour after meals.

- Avoid crash diets, fad diets, fasting, diet pills and diets with very low calories.

- Do not hurry, worry, hate, lie, detest, negate, cringe and laze.

The Dos of a Healthy Routine

- Eat food in small quantities at regular intervals.

- Address your food weaknesses (chocolate, ice cream, soft drinks etc) and overcome them successfully.

- Drink lots of water.

- Start a meal with lots of salads of all varieties.

- Consume RDA of protein and complex carbohydrates.

- Eat at least one fruit every day. Preferably citrus.

- Exercise at least one hour every day (this includes gym, aerobics and flexibility training).

- Read, write, think, play, work, laugh, pray, trust, help, meditate, reaffirm life and search, find, explore and enhance the inner rhythm of your life.

Wellness

We can now say that we are fully equipped with total knowledge about obesity, health and fitness. Now let us think about wellness. High level of wellness clearly goes beyond optimum physical fitness and absence of disease. Wellness incorporates fitness with additional dimensions of life, nutrition, stress management, disease prevention, social support, nurturance (sense of being needed), spirituality, personal safety, substance control, physical exam, health education and environmental support.

The seven dimensions of wellness are physical fitness, emotional fitness, intellectual fitness, spiritual fitness, environmental fitness, occupational fitness and social fitness.

Emotional fitness: Like physical fitness, your emotional fitness is also one of the dimensions of wellness. Try to improve your emotional quotient. It teaches you to understand and respect the emotional feelings of others, so that even you feel satisfied.

Intellectual fitness: Try to improve your intellectual fitness. Be keen on improving knowledge. When you are reading, surfing the internet or exploring any other media, you are updating your knowledge. Knowledge is the base of personality. Keep learning something new at regular intervals, to keep your brain active. Deeper your knowledge in any field, the more meaningful is your personality and life.

Spiritual fitness: If you are spiritual and believe that God or some supernatural power has an influence on your life, you believe that doing good for others is good for yourself. Spirituality helps manage stress and gives peace. You can then rely on this power during crisis.

Environmental fitness: Creating and maintaining a good environment within yourself, within your family, within your society and globally will protect you and the world. Be aware of the environment, create it, maintain it and protect it. It will then protect you and maintain you. It will also offer good health and quality of life.

Occupational fitness: Try to select an occupation of your liking, otherwise start liking your occupation. Overcome occupational health and other hazards. Be satisfied with what you can earn and try for higher progress in your occupation. Give your 100% efforts and you will get 100% from your occupation.

Social fitness: Now plan your social fitness. Build healthy relations. Maintain them. Do not compete, do not hate. Do not even think anything bad about anybody. Help and love others. Do not expect anything in return. Try to help society with your capabilities like knowledge, money and work. Listen to the problems of other people. Reaffirm life. Search, find and explore positive things.

With all these dimensions in place, along with physical fitness and good nutrition, you can build health and wellness.

Life is wonderful for you now! Live life to its fullest potential with fullest quality!

Muscles of the body.

Glossary

Adenosine triphosphate: The high energy phosphate molecule that provides energy for cellular function

Anabolic steroids: A synthetic version of the male sex hormone testosterone, which promotes muscle development and hypertrophy

Angiogenesis: Capillary (blood vessel) formation into a tumor

Atherosclerosis: Fatty/cholesterol deposits in the walls of arteries, leading to formation of plaque

Benign: Non-cancerous

Beta carotene: A precursor to vitamin A

Catabolism: Any destructive process by which complex substances are converted into more simple compounds by Jiving cells

Chronic obstructive pulmonary disease (COPD): Diseases that limit air flow to the lungs

Concentric muscle contraction: A dynamic contraction in which the muscle shortens as it develops tension

Cognitions: Current thoughts or feelings that can function as antecedents or consequences for overt behavior

Deoxyribonucleic acid (DNA): Genetic substance with which genes are made up; a molecule that bears the cell's genetic code

Diastolic blood pressure: Pressure exerted by the blood against the walls of the arteries during the relaxation phase (diastole) of the heart.

Diuretics: Medications that produce an increase in urine volume and sodium exertion

Homocysteine: Intermediate amino acid in the interconversion of two other amino acids: methionine and cysteine

Hypercholesterolemia: Excess cholesterol in the blood

Contact

Status Health Club Pvt Ltd Pune
791/216 Bhandarkar Road,
Deccan Gymkhana, Pune - 411 004
Phone: 020–25675070
sumedha.fitness@gmail.com
www.statushealthclub.com